What People are saying about Don't Leave Momma Home With The Dog:

Anyone caring for a person with dementia will find hope and healing in <u>Don't Leave Momma Home With The Dog</u>.
Jo Huey, a professional speaker and author of two books on caregiving, shares her journey from a personal and professional perspective. When Jo, a twenty-year expert in the field, fell into the pits of guilt and despair in dealing with her mother with rapidly declining dementia, she was forced to learn and practice her own lessons. Her heartfelt story shares triumphs, frustrations, pains and privileges while offering new tools and skills, easing the caregiver's journey.
LeAnn Thieman
coauthor *Chicken Soup for the Caregiver's Soul*

"This is an incredible book written by an incredible lady. Jo Huey takes her readers on a heartfelt journey of understanding dementia and how to minimize its impact on the person with the disease, and the caregiver, in particular. It is written with great sensitivity and warmth. <u>Don't Leave Momma Home With The Dog,</u> is a must for anyone caring for a loved one facing Alzheimer's disease or related dementia."
Dick Bruso
Founder of Heard Above The Noise

Don't Leave Momma Home With The Dog

Why Caregivers Do What They Do!

Jo Huey

Author of Alzheimer's Disease: Help and Hope

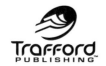

Trafford
PUBLISHING™

Editor - Virginia Vehaskari, PhD www.gveditingassociates.com
Book Cover/Designer - Maria K. Bell www.mariabelliimages.com
Photographer - Randall Miller Randall's Photography www.randallsphoto.com

Note for Librarians: A cataloguing record for this book is available from Library
and Archives Canada at www.collectionscanada.ca/amicus/index-e.html

Printed in Victoria, BC, Canada.

ISBN: 978-1-4251-2705-3

*We at Trafford believe that it is the responsibility of us all, as both individuals
and corporations, to make choices that are environmentally and socially sound.
You, in turn, are supporting this responsible conduct each time you purchase a
Trafford book, or make use of our publishing services. To find out how you are
helping, please visit www.trafford.com/responsiblepublishing.html*

*Our mission is to efficiently provide the world's finest, most comprehensive
book publishing service, enabling every author to experience success.
To find out how to publish your book, your way, and have it available
worldwide, visit us online at www.trafford.com/10510*

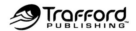

www.trafford.com

North America & international
toll-free: 1 888 232 4444 (USA & Canada)
phone: 250 383 6864 ♦ fax: 250 383 6804
email: info@trafford.com

The United Kingdom & Europe
phone: +44 (0)1865 722 113 ♦ local rate: 0845 230 9601
facsimile: +44 (0)1865 722 868 ♦ email: info.uk@trafford.com

10 9 8 7 6 5 4 3 2

Dedication

I dedicate this book to the memory of my dear father whom I often discussed in the book. Obviously, it is also dedicated to my dear mother who has continued to support and teach me even in her infirmity. I am so blessed to have had such wonderful parents.

Acknowledgement

Special thanks to my editor Dr. Virginia Vehaskari. Without her persistent and consistent assistance, this book would never have been completed.

Thank you so much to my daughter Jenae and son Jason for their support and assistance since Hurricane Katrina so completely devastated my life.

Table of Contents

Introduction

In this book I am sharing with you how, as a professional with almost 20 years of experience in the field of 24-hour care for persons with dementia, and with over a decade of support group facilitation, I fell into the same pits of guilt and despair of dealing with a mother with rapidly declining Vascular Dementia, just as if I had no training or experience at all.

Giving advice about what to do as a caregiver for a person with Dementia (regardless of whether it is caused from Alzheimer's, Vascular or from some other disease process) had been my life work for nearly 20 years. I designed and taught a communication tool, The Ten Absolutes, wrote a book Alzheimer's Disease: Help and Hope, gave presentations all over the country, trained professional caregivers, counseled families and offered them solutions for everything from giving a bath to how and when to plan for Day Care and Long Term Care. I not only believed the things I taught, but actually did them; I could give a bath to the most difficult person and I could engage any person with dementia. However, when something appeared to be wrong with my own mother, I denied its existence, ignored all the signs, did all the wrong things, and allowed myself to become burned out. I waited too long to not let her live alone and to place her in Day Care. Worst of all even after she was living with me I was still leaving her alone enough to actually put her in "Harms Way" for I Left Her "Home With The Dog." I should have reported myself to Elderly Protective Services.

I believe I made these errors in judgment for the same reason the majority of people do. I wanted to protect her from embarrassment. I did not want her to have a debilitating disease; I wanted to take care of her myself and most of all I wanted to give back to her just a little of what she had so unselfishly given to me. What I learned from these mistakes is very apparent if you will read this and the previous paragraph—there are too many I's. When it comes to taking care of someone with Dementia, the first thing you must embrace is- IT IS NOT ABOUT YOU AND WHAT YOU WANT—It is about him or her. What they really need is a protected life with a safe environment, where they have friends, peers, where they feel useful and each day has purpose. They need to be loved, just as they are, and they need to be enjoyed, and not pitied by those who love them. They can have this good life and if you can concentrate on how to make that life for them, the journey will be less arduous not only for you but especially for them.

Writing this book has been a mixed blessing. Sometimes it has been just too difficult and I have wrestled with sharing so much of my life and especially sharing my mother's life. However, if it can assist others in this journey then it is worth the pain. I wrestled with the format of how to tell the story without whining too much or looking so bad when I was such a horrible caregiver. See, I still think 'It is about me' at least sometimes! I finally decided to create a new Ten Absolutes and this again is for Caregivers. The difference is that this one tells you what to do for yourself not what to do for the person with dementia. I decided to write this book like my first book and use one of the ten absolutes for each chapter. At the beginning of each chapter I am giving information about that absolute. Then in the second part of the chapter I am telling our story, from my perspective, with which you might identify. Then for the wrap-up, there will be two sections, one of privilege and one of pain. Both sections help you make your choice of whether you want to take this journey with privilege or with pain. I learned that the choice is yours. It is very much like the old adage of looking at a cup half-empty or a cup half full. Your perception of the cup is the determining factor. The amount of liquid in the cup does not change. The journey is much the same and it can be a long journey, however, you can choose how to travel on this journey.

In no way do I want to minimize the devastation this disease causes for the person with the disease and also for everyone who cares about them. Most diseases are horrible and devastating—but this disease is what it is and unfortunately, we are not offered any options. It is my wish that in sharing with you my pain and contrasting the pain with the privilege, your journey will be easier and you can make wiser choices. For those of you who still feel guilty or regret the choices you made, this book might provide you with some closure or anesthesia to reduce that pain until it is manageable. If you find yourself in the muck of pain and misery, you can just regroup and accept the privilege. You can't change history but you can be forgiven and that usually is just a matter of forgiving yourself. You also can change your approach today so you don't sentence yourself to "living with regret".

1

Never Assume Always Examine

Never Assume: It is critical to get your affairs in order, e.g. long-term care insurance, wills, and power of attorney and then get a complete examination. Don't let fear or assumption prevent you from the care you deserve.

Always Examine: Dementia, whether it is caused from Alzheimer's disease, Vascular or from some other illness is a diagnosis of "rule out". It is critical that you make certain, with an extensive examination, so the appropriate treatment or reversal can be addressed as early as possible.

Now What Does That Mean?

Usually in the course of this disease the person who has the disease early on states, "There must be something wrong with me because, I keep getting lost, I keep losing everything and I can't even remember people that I have known for a long time." To which their family and friends reply, "Oh, that happens to everyone, don't worry about it you are probably just stressed". Then as the symptoms progress the person with the disease knows something is wrong and it is so frightening that they begin to hide the symptoms. Their friends and family start asking questions of each other, such as, "Did you notice how many times she told us about her friend's party; did she tell you that she lost her car the other day and took a taxi home; does it seem like he/she is withdrawing from the group?" Eventually, it is so obvious to all that something is wrong, then the person with the disease is busy hiding it for their own self-preservation and the family and friends are hiding it to protect their loved one. Everyone hopes it is a mistake and tomorrow it will "go away" and their lives can get back to normal.

It is not easy to get a diagnosis but it is important and a complete work-up, not just an opinion, is very necessary. There are differing opinions about what a complete work-up is and this book is not giving medical advice. It is important that you seek medical advice and that you follow the protocol of a good memory disorder center recommendation for this exam. It is also necessary that you feel confident that the diagnostic procedure was thorough enough that you feel the diagnosis is accurate and reliable. Your denial will provide you with enough opportunity to question during this journey. It is critical that you not just accept the opinion of one person or just assume that they have Alzheimer's.

It is so important to have a complete work-up early on when anyone exhibits problems of being able to function in their every day lives. The diagnostic process for dementia symptoms (regardless of their cause) is one of "rule out" which means doctors can successfully "rule out" anything that is treatable. The medications that treat the symptoms of dementia are more effective the earlier they are used in the course of the disease. I have been telling people this professionally on a daily basis for over a decade so why did I wait so long to have my mother diagnosed? Part of it was denial but another part is what caregivers so often face, persons who do know the person well, and often some who do not, have difficulty seeing anything wrong. My Mom's geriatrician and a dear friend of mine a neuro-psychologist, who does diagnostic testing for Alzheimer's disease, felt that the testing was unnecessary. I think the reason was that my mother was socially so adept and generally so pleasant that it was just hard to believe that there was really anything wrong with her.

The other thing that was a part of my mother's work-up that was so important was they did occupational therapy testing. This testing has the person with the disease go through the mechanics of taking a bath, getting the water ready, going through each step of what to do next. It also includes the mechanics of preparing a cup of tea and selecting clothing for certain situations. There is a test available (only a few insurances cover this test and it can be expensive) that test to see if the person with the disease is capable of driving safely. The importance of this testing is that it determines whether the person with the disease should live alone, or if it is safe for them to be driving.

In retrospect, not having Mom tested/diagnosed until 2004, though she already lived with me, was the first time I truly let my caregiver status cloud my judgment as a professional. It certainly was not the last!

Our story—from my perspective!

You can't change history. It doesn't really matter if you "should have known" or "probably knew for a long time," that your loved one had something going on that made them different from the way they once were. What does matter is that you have a complete medical examination to address the dementia symptoms or the concerns that you have with challenges of your loved one who is continuing to exist in their everyday life patterns.

When a loved one has a dementia, (whether it is caused from Alzheimer's disease, Vascular or some other disease process) eventually we hear ourselves saying something like this, "He/She was actually diagnosed 3 years ago, but if we look back, now we can see that the symptoms had started long before."

When you are a Caregiver of a person with a dementia you need to become familiar with the definition of Denial, which from a psychological perspective, "Is a state of mind marked by a refusal or an inability to recognize and deal with a serious personal problem." The reason you need to actually have this term defined is because you and most everyone who knows the person with the disease are going to spend most of their time in denial. There is little comfort for you when your loved one receives a dementia diagnosis. The only immediate protection for your loved one and thus yourself is to bask in denial whenever possible. There are many reasons for this psychological phenomenon and I truly believe it is a form of self-preservation. No one wants to have to face a loved one presenting with Alzheimer's disease, one of the most dreaded and difficult diseases possible.

This is how the story went with my mother and me. My sister had been telling me for at least a year that something was really wrong with Mom and she couldn't stay at home any more. I told her that I talked to Mom every night and she seemed alright to me. DENIAL!

Let me tell you our story. I've been single most of my adult life. Because I was the only child in my family who was single, I spent more time with my parents than my siblings. I spent an inordinate amount of time with my Mother after my dad died in 1993. I called her every day after dad died and whenever I could, I would take her traveling with me, mostly to my daughter's out of state home. Mom was always afraid of heights but she truly wasn't afraid to fly if she were with me. I would talk her into coming to stay at my house, but there had to be a reason for her to come because she loved to be in her own home. So, I would tell her that I needed her to help me with a project, usually moving, painting, or taking care of the dog.

Then I learned something more about my Mom and how she let me be independent. I made a huge lifestyle change in 1997 and agreed to move across the country to New Orleans. Mom didn't discourage me but often after I moved when I would call her, still every day, she would sound so sad. I would ask her what was wrong and she would say, "I just miss you". I realized then that she had a really hard time adjusting to my being far away but she had never said any thing against my moving. I think probably, if I am being honest, it was also the start of her physical and mental decline. So, I would have her come and stay with me really often. She spent a lot of time in New Orleans with me. I was very busy and I would take her with me whenever I could. However, on days I couldn't, when there were long days I would apologize for leaving her alone so long. She would say, "At home, I am always alone, here I am only alone until you get home so it is better." But, eventually she would say, "I have to go home to my house" and so I would find a way to get her back to her own home. The first time she came to stay, she flew with my sister and brother-in-law and she had to fly home alone. Thank heaven it was before September 11, 2001. I can never remember being so worried as when I put her on that plane, I went all the way into the plane with her because I knew she was so scared to fly alone. She did just fine and my sister got her directly off the plane, but I avoided her flying alone if at all possible. She flew to my home so often, all my friends and business associates got to know her.

In 2001 we were going to Hawaii to my daughters wedding and Mom and I were so excited about going to Hawaii. However, a week before we went she got the results of her blood tests from a Senior Fair. My brother-in-law was volunteering at the Senior Fair and had insisted that my Mom go have her blood tested. Mom was rarely sick and consequently did not go to the doctor. My family, with the exception of me, who had worked primarily in the medical field, felt that going to doctors was only if you were really ill. Prevention was staying away from doctors and just not going. Mom's blood tests were awful! They showed serious liver problems—in fact, they showed over 20 things wrong and had a notice with instructions to call her doctor immediately. Mom decided that she could just call the doctor after she got home from Hawaii and oddly enough I agreed. My sister, who never goes to the doctor, totally disagreed and she called the doctor. They told her that Mom should stop taking the anti-cholesterol medication she had been on for several years and come in as soon as she returned from Hawaii.

Apparently, she always cancelled or forgotten the doctor appointments to have her routine blood checks.

That was the beginning of Mom's bad health journey. The doctor sent her to specialists and they decided after much testing, all of which she responded to very poorly, showed that she had a serious liver problem. In all of this testing and questioning, and answering, we discovered that she had been eating very poorly, which was the reason she had lost so much weight. When I called her every night she always told me what she had cooked and eaten that day and apparently most of that was confabulation—though I still believed it for at least another year! My sister was run ragged with the entire doctor appointments, monitoring medications that Mom usually refused (probably forgot) to take and her continued downward spiraling health problems. When my sister would talk about Mom's health to me I would assure her that there was really nothing that wrong with Mom. I told my sister that she just was just looking for things to worry about.

In 2002, Mom turned 80 and my sister was insisting then that Mom couldn't live alone. Though, I was the expert, I insisted that she seemed alright when I called her every night and she was just fine when she stayed with me. Somehow I didn't notice that she was no longer trying to have dinner ready when I got home and she was so glad to see me when I got there. I kept remembering the previous times and just wasn't paying attention to the changes—I think they call that denial!! She continued to have serious health problems, some as a result of the medication she was taking for the liver condition and she continued having weight loss. When she would stay with me, she would be fine and we increased those times, yet when she went home, she would spiral downward again quite rapidly. I was still in denial.

When my sister called to insist that Mom shouldn't live alone any more I knew it wasn't a problem, I would take care of her. I brought her home with me to assess the situation. My sister was right; Mom had declined very rapidly even since her last visit. For the first time in the last six years she was not particularly happy to be at my house; she kept telling me she was not going to stay. I tried to tell her that we needed to discuss what she wanted to do with her life because living alone didn't seem to be working. She didn't want to discuss it. She became seriously ill. We went to the emergency room and I saw how frightened she was. She told me she could not stay in the hospital alone. Fortunately, she did not have to be admitted to the hospital. She had some fairly significant health problems but they were all easily addressed with medications. She started taking the medications and they actually helped her but all she wanted to do was get well enough to go home. I kept trying to discuss what she wanted to do in the future but what she wanted to do was to not discuss the subject. I gave her options including me moving back home and living with her, but she didn't want to discuss anything about her life. She did get better and she decided that all she wanted to do was go home, go to her high school reunion, get her house painted, and live happily ever after. I was so stressed; I didn't know what on earth to do, because the more I tried to discuss the subject, the less she would discuss it. She just kept saying things like, "I don't know why everyone thinks I am sick, I feel just fine. They are making me sick."

She was with me for 2 months and they were the most difficult months in our relationship of over 50 years. We never even had difficulties when I was a teenager. But now it seemed like we were always on a "different page" and no matter what I said, it seemed to make her uncomfortable. I couldn't imagine what had happened to my sweet, cheerful, amicable mother. When we went to see her doctor before going home she happily told her that she was going home. When the doctor asked her when she was coming back, she said that she would return in a year because she only visited once a year. The doctor was as shocked as I was and said, "Well I need to see you sooner than that." Mom said, "Well I'll just have to go to my old doctor, because I only visit once a year." I tried to discuss this with Mom and told her she had always come every month or two for a few weeks and she said, "No, I only visit once a year. I will be back next year." I just wanted to cry, I didn't seem to be able to do anything to make her more comfortable and I couldn't move to her home without some planning that would take me at least a year. I had thought she would just stay with me and make frequent trips home, however, all she wanted to do was go home and come back in a year.

Within a few months her doctor (whom she had gone to for years) pointed out to Mom in front of me, "Helen, it seems that when you are with Jo you are fine, but when you are home you seem to not do so well." So, my denial couldn't be denied and I took Mom home with me to stay with the intent that I would "wrap up" what I was doing and move back and live with her. She had always wanted me to come home. When I got divorced in 1976, she wanted my children and me to move home. When dad died in 1993, she wanted me to move home. Now it looked like I needed to move home. However, I just couldn't seem to get things to work for me to move home and I really tried. I tried to find work there that would compliment what

I was doing and things just didn't work out; it was as if that wasn't supposed to happen. In May 2003, Mom's heart really started on a decline. When she had, what we thought was a mild heart attack. As it turned out the doctors realized that she had really serious heart problems and then we began all the extensive medications to fix her heart. She initially refused all the medications and was for the first time in my life often angry with me. First, I wouldn't let her go home and then I made her take all her medicine which actually was the medicine that had made her ill in the first place. Now she was only going to get worse which made it so much harder for me. For the first time in my life, I was fighting with my mother. The only thing that had changed was that she was actually saying what she thought—which as an expert should have been a clue. But, no, it took Mom to tell me that she really had some problems with early dementia!

Finally, in August of 2004 I actually had Mom evaluated for dementia and it should have been no surprise to me that she clearly had dementia of the Vascular Type and all indications were that she needed 24-hour supervision and she was not safe to be left alone. By then she had already been living with me for nearly two years, though unhappily, and until then I was still trying to have her make the decisions for her life, of which she was not capable. However, even as the expert, I in no way followed my own advice. Had I just had her evaluated earlier I would have known that there "was something wrong with her" and we could have had a better 20 months.

This is exactly what this chapter is about—we can't change history, but we can learn from it. Looking forward is the only option. If you are someone who is struggling with a diagnosis, struggle no longer—Make the Appointment!

Pain or Privilege?

There is truly nothing more wonderful than having a family. Now my family wasn't "Leave it to Beaver" it was more like "All in the Family" but with more children. My dad acted like Archie Bunker but he truly was a pillar of strength; he cared deeply and made a real contribution to our society and to the lives of his children. Not unlike Edith, my Mom was socialized to do what she was told and she did it and embraced it because it was truly her calling in life.

Regardless of the family dynamics, good or bad, perfect or devastating, real or imagined, when it comes to families it seems inherent in each of us to one day deal with the loss of family members: grandparents, parents, aunts & uncles, siblings, spouses and for some even children.

It is a well-known psychological fact that loss brings pain. Once again, regardless of our relationship or history with the person, the loss requires dealing with something that brings pain. As a society, we don't seem to do real well at acknowledging this pain or dealing with the pain. I lost my dad to a long painful cancer death and it was devastating. I have spent 20 years working with families of persons with Alzheimer's disease or a related dementia and their pain is equally or maybe even more devastating. With the brain degeneration illness, what seems to be the most devastating is that it lasts so long. Because of the length of the illness and the afflicted person's inability to make decisions or care for themselves, it requires family involvement. Members of families sometimes often choose to be uninvolved and while that creates a lot of ire on the part of other family members or friends of the afflicted, at the time it is not necessarily the least painful route. It is not at all unusual to encounter persons who painfully tell you the story of their loved one, whom they couldn't or didn't see any more because they didn't know them anyway. In my experience, this is the person who suffers the most. They experience guilt, which by definition is "wrongdoing accompanied by feelings of regret and shame."

Now, I will attempt to explain the privilege part of this book. In response to the laments of the caregivers, in support groups, I have often said with "tongue in cheek", that all they ever got from family and friends was criticism. Instead, I told them that they should just consider it their privilege to have the responsibility of the loved one. While the comment was made to make them feel better, and it did, it was laced with sarcasm. However, I think that very term became a real tool for me in dealing with the loss of my mother. The old saying, "Hindsight is 20-20 vision," was a special gift for me. Because of the unplanned move created by Hurricane Katrina, I lost the choice of where my mother should live. My family, for the first time, instead of saying it was my issue as it was my "bailiwick," determined that Mom would be better off back in her home town especially because there was a home there that she could afford and could meet her needs. However, that was not where I lived and so I lost the "privilege" of being her primary caregiver and in fact I became a long distance caregiver. While, I haven't handed out criticism about what the relatives have or haven't done, I have felt the loss of being the primary caregiver and thus realize that it truly was a privilege. I want to share, the privilege I had even in the toughest of circumstances, to be my mother's caregiver. It was truly my privilege. My fantasy, every day, though I know my mother is well cared for, happy and content, is that I can bring her back to live with me so I can be with her for the last days of her life.

The most difficult part of this journey is to not have that privilege. In a world of self-absorption and "me-ism" I have to tell myself daily—"It isn't about me, but it is about her and what is best for her." That is the real theme of this book, how to make it about them, how to make it for them, how to do things for them and not to them. In case I haven't made myself clear, because it is a truly hard concept, the sooner you can make it about them, not you—the better it gets for you! That concept just does not make sense but it is true! That is what is so difficult about this disease.

One of my dearest friends of all time, a gentleman who lived a truly exemplary life, always said in support groups. Remember, "You are doing this for them, not to them". It is so true and because it is the wisdom I have to use every day in the end days of this journey, I wish for you to use that phrase too. I dedicate this book to that great man, Paul Stall, for the wisdom he imparted that will truly help us all.

So, as you read this book I, as the author, am giving you the opportunity for it to be, "All about you". The pain is yours, the privilege is yours, and there in lies my sarcasm. However, the choices you make must be, "for them, not to them," and that is the most difficult part of this long journey. It can be painful but if you can shift from pain to privilege, the pain will truly subside and we can continue to improve the inevitable part of life that we as a society so carefully ignore—the end of life, be it a long journey or not!

2

Never Justify
Always Authorize

Never Justify: There is no realistic way to justify what must be done for a person with dementia, regardless of the cause for the dementia it is an illness. Illness changes the status-quo. Your responsibility is to take care of them the best you know how. You are the person responsible. Other people will always have opinions but you have the responsibility.

Always Authorize: You have the authority and you need to accept the authority for the decisions that need to be made. Your loved one is not in a position to make these decisions, unless it is a very early diagnosis. Do not expect them to make the decisions that are best and do not expect their blessings. They chose you to be responsible so you must be responsible. This is the most difficult for spouses, but you promised "in sickness or in health" and you have to keep that promise. It is also difficult to make decisions for a parent because it is a role reversal. Illness changes things and it is difficult for everyone.

Now What Does That Mean?

'Aging in Place' is a buzzword in long-term care. It is really a buzzword for elder advocates who are against "institutionalization" or "warehousing", a more graphic term for institutionalization. However, like most buzzwords it really is not clearly defined and can be misused to each person's disadvantage.

Let us discuss 'Aging in Place':

Home: How do we really define it? Why does the word carry such power? There are plenty of statistics that tell us that everyone, elderly in particular, want to be "home" rather than any other place. Is it something that is overblown? Is it something that is good for them? Can home be a state of mind and can that state of mind be changed?

Is "home" bricks and sticks, furniture or a patio, familiarity, a neighborhood? Can you take those things with you? Could "home" merely represent a more comfortable better place in time? Can "home" be created anywhere if a person is well cared for, entertained, feel they belong, and not lonely? Does it mean something different to different people? How and who should determine when "home" is no longer the appropriate place.

When does safety come into the picture? Is aging in place something that has been created in the marketplace; does the term have different meaning to different people?

I believe "home" to my mother meant, pride, the place that belonged to her, that she had to protect, that had familiar things, responsibility, and safety. However, in the past few years it had also meant loneliness, fear, and maybe even danger. Being in her actual home had resulted in her weight loss, tears, and confabulation (telling people what she thought they wanted to hear when she did not know the answers to their questions).

Is there a way to blend all of these things to create a win/win situation or do we have to stay with the past idea that there comes a time when you cannot and should not stay home alone? Should there be an option for someone to stay with you? Is there a set of criteria that helps with that decision or should it be as individual as each individual.

These questions probably have many answers but some of the questions that will make the answers easier might be as follows:

Review what your loved one has said in the past—Did they really ask you to always let them stay in their home, to never "put them someplace," or is that just what we all assume we have heard. My mother never asked me to make that promise, did yours? What did your parents or spouse do with their parents? My Mom had my grandfather live with her for only a few weeks. When she discovered he had let a stranger into their home, she arranged to place him in a nursing home. I must have made that hard for her because I offered to let him come and live with me instead. If it was hard, she didn't show it, she never even considered my offer. She found a place close to her and she put him there. He never really seemed to mind and she never seemed distressed about the decision. She did faithfully visit him and tried to address his every need.

Has anything been put in writing? If your loved one has appointed someone to make decisions, do you know what made that decision? I know that my sister encouraged my Mom to make those decisions but it was clearly Mom's wishes, she made certain that I was on the paperwork and she had my brother put on for financial decisions after her death. Do you know your family history and the role each person played? Who would your loved one trust to make the decisions and is that decision maker involved now? Why did your loved one appoint a particular person to make these decisions? It may be difficult as a family member to understand that decision, especially if that person is not you or the one you would have chosen. Is that person, even if they were the favorite, more likely to make the decisions that the loved one would have made if they were still able to do so?

Is there a person who does not want to be a part of the decision making process? Is there a person who disagrees with whatever decision is being made and are they being argumentative or really assessing all the possibilities? What would truly happen if that person took over? Is it more appropriate for someone to have an extended visit in the home of the person for whom you are concerned, would it be possible for that person of concern to visit one or all of the children for an extended period of time?

Who determines what is really safe? Do you wait until there is a disaster or do you evaluate and then accept the evaluation? Did you know there is an entire classification of person whose job it is to make such assessments? They are called Geriatric Care Managers and they are available all over the country. They are professionals with the knowledge and credentials to evaluate all of these situations. They are not free, though some long-term care insurance policies may cover some of their fees. However, they are the best investment any family can make to determine the real situation. If there is dis-agreement after the assessment is received, it should be treated like a medical opinion or a bid for work to be done. Have 2 or 3 other people do the same assessment and compare the results. You will be amazed at the consistency in their information. By the time an eval-uation is needed, the need will be obvious. The other advantage of having such an assessment is that it prevents many family squabbles and allows you to truly make decisions for the person whose brain is degenerating. It also prevents the fear of doing something too soon or waiting until disaster strikes to make decisions.

Our story—from my perspective!

As I confessed in Chapter 1 for the first time in my life, my mother and I were in disagreement and often. I just wanted her to make decisions; no, actually I wanted her to agree with what I thought was best for her and I wanted her not only to agree with me I wanted her to give me her blessings on that agreement. All I was asking was for her to decide to completely change her life and to choose that option as if it were really a choice. She couldn't live alone anymore, for pure physical reasons because I was in too much denial to accept any other reasons or to even have the necessary work-up that I would have recommended to any with whom I worked profes-sionally. In retrospect, I think that I didn't want to acknowledge the difficulty of making decisions for someone else, especially a parent. I didn't want to face the fact that our roles had changed and she was no longer the mother and I was no longer the daughter. I got so caught up in wanting to allow her to be the parent that I was neglecting her capabilities. This is the rule not the exception for caregivers of persons with dementia symptoms—why should I be different? Could it have been because I counseled persons, very effectively, on this very subject all the time?

So, for many months, Mom and I were quite miserable and our conversations were repeatedly as follows:

I like staying with you but if I do, "they" will sell my house. "Mom, who do you think they are?" I ask in exasperation. "Besides, so what if the house is sold, if you are staying with me why do you care about the house?"

"I can't stay with you forever, you will want to send me home and I won't have anyplace to go!" she replied.

I cannot imagine that I would ever have wanted her to go home and even if I did, she could not stay home anymore. The guilt just would not let me go.

I had many a pity party! I just did not understand why I had to make the decisions. I didn't understand why she wouldn't make the decisions that were best for her. I needed to go and live with her, which is what she really wanted. Even if I had to work in a different field for a few years, it should have been o.k. I needed to make plans and go and I tried. I tried many things but it just did not work out. Maybe I didn't want it badly enough. I did want it for her but not for me. I had always thought of myself as a city girl and I really loved living in the city of New Orleans. Mom loved it there too so why didn't we just settle down and live there.

For the first time in our lives we were really at odds. We would go along just fine and then I would start questioning her and trying to get her to make decisions. Not just decisions but the decisions I deemed best for her. She usually never made decisions because dad always handled that so why was I forcing the issue. I just didn't want the responsibility and I didn't really feel it my place to make the decisions. I don't know who I thought should make the decisions. My sister and I had Mom's Power of Attorney and my sister was in agreement that she needed to not be alone. Mom had signed the power of attorney so why did I think that she should make the decisions.

Maybe I just needed to let her go home and soon she would see for herself that being at home alone wasn't working out and she would make the decision, to come and live permanently with me. Now, we had already tried that for a long time before and we already knew the answer. How on earth could I even consider such a solution? Yet, it went through my mind all the time.

We boarded the plane to go home and on the plane she asked me something and I gave her what I thought was a reasonable answer. She looked at me and said, "Why don't you use your stuff on me?" I asked her, "What stuff are you talking about." She said, "See that is what I mean, you argue with me about everything; you know the stuff you teach to other people." The "stuff" Mom was referring to is the Ten Absolutes I developed for caregivers of persons with Alzheimer's disease. I said, "But, Mom, that is for caregivers of people with dementia and you don't have dementia." She replied, "You could be nice to me anyway." I was absolutely floored but then I began to laugh, mostly at myself because I realized that I had clearly forgotten to use "my stuff" just as she had so appropriately accused me. I was so concerned about being a caregiver that I forgot to just treat her as I always had, as my fun-loving Mom. She wasn't feeling well and I was so concerned about making her well and including her in plans for her future that I forgot about the person she had always been. My Mom never liked to make decisions; her decisions were all made by my dad. She had never been sick and she didn't take medicine. She had loved to visit with me because we did fun things and she wasn't lonely. Recently, we had only talked about decisions she had to make, visited doctors, had tests and had taken medicine; we did fewer fun things because we were too busy and too tired. But most of all we didn't enjoy the pleasure of each other's company and it was because I was trying too hard. Wow! What an eye opener! What a Revelation! I was the one who had changed and she was responding to the changes in me.

Shocking! I did not know if I could hang on to the thought that, she did not want to discuss or make decisions! I didn't know if I could just make the decisions, present them nicely, not take offense or try to explain when she didn't agree. This is exactly what I had been telling people to do for years but I was not following my own advice!

Did you notice here that I was still not accepting that she had any problems other than the physical ones and I was not even thinking about having a work-up to address her Dementia symptoms? In my caregiver denial I was not taking care of her in the way that I as a professional knew to be the best way to care for her.

So I tried to do better and we began to enjoy each other a lot more but I also noticed many changes in both of us. For me there was more stress and for her there was an increasing need for attention and assistance.

I'd always told caregivers of persons with Alzheimer's disease that when they found themselves gritting their teeth, clenching their fists and losing their cool over little things they needed to regroup. They needed to regroup for themselves, not for the person for whom they were caring. It was also a sign that the caregivers's were placing themselves in a situation for serious burnout and that they needed to start doing less and start getting help. They always said there was no help available and that was absolutely not true. My response has always been, "There is help available; one just has to be willing to ask for it, accept it when it is offered and not expect it to be, as good as we do". Now that I had become the caregiver for my mother I realized that I needed to "listen to my own advice." That was not an easy thing to do.

I worked all day with people in need. It was my job to oversee the day to day management of an assisted living community for persons with Alzheimer's disease. In addition, I worked with the families of our residents, prospective families, facilitated several support groups, spoke, taught and trained family, and professional caregivers on effective communication. I was on the podium, phone, or with people all day. When I got home, I loved the fact that my dog did not talk. I loved absolute quiet, did not even turn on the radio or television, screened my calls and only took the most important calls, as I just had to regroup to avoid burnout. My life had changed as I now had my mother staying with me or I was monitoring her closely or at a distance when she was staying at her home. Ultimately, I was segueing into living with her full time, probably at her home as she truly should not be alone any longer.

When I got home now she greeted me with, "I thought you would be here sooner" and initially I found myself being very defensive and saying, "I told you I would be home about 6:00 and it is only 5:45". She immediately said, "I am just glad you are here," and I would immediately realize that she had been lonely. I usually walked the dog and sat and drank something and often ignored dinner altogether. Later, I might eat something like popcorn or cereal or meet friends for dinner if they called and wanted to go out. I usually read or worked on some project and tried to go to bed early. However, now Mom wanted to hear about my day, wanted to know if the dog did any good while he is out, wanted to know if we were going to call my siblings and what we are having for dinner.

I have always jokingly referred to this time of day as "sundowning." Sundowning is a term that many professionals use to describe escalation of adverse behaviors of persons with Alzheimer's disease late in the day. I have always described this as being the most difficult time of day in most households and recount how difficult this time of day was in my own home for years, especially when I had two small children and had worked all day. I am of the opinion that if you don't do something well the first time you always get the opportunity to try it again. Apparently, it was my time to try again, with my mother's need for my undivided attention I had the opportunity to practice. Maybe this time I could do better!

I actually wrote the paragraph above for an article but still neglected to have my mother evaluated for her symptoms. Fortunately, I did have the good sense to identify the next symptoms and I did something about them. It was not long until one day I came home and she told me, "It is a good thing you got here, Cezar (our 125 lb. dog) and I were just getting ready to go and find you, and I heard a siren and just knew you were in an accident." This scared me to death and I immediately began looking for an apartment where we would no longer be on the street so she could actually get out and get lost. In addition, I realized that I could no longer leave her alone all day. Yes, I should have realized I could no longer leave her alone at all, however, that would clearly not fit into our lifestyle so I didn't think that far!

Fortunately, for me, I knew all the resources in New Orleans and I called my dear friend at the Uptown Shepherd Center and told her I would like Mom to come and be a volunteer at the center. I told her of my concerns about Mom being alone all day and worrying about me and possibly going out to look for me. I was still in total denial. She knew my Mom and said she would be delighted to let her come and they really needed someone to answer the phone and Mom would be great at that.

Then I made yet another mistake I discussed it with my mother and even arranged to take her on an interview. Mom said she wasn't interested but would go with me because she liked my friends. I took her on Friday and she visited with everyone and after we left she told me it just wasn't the place for her and she wasn't going back. Now I had really backed myself into a corner because she had to go back because I couldn't leave her alone all day. So on Monday morning I got her ready to go, she didn't mind because she loved to go with me. However, when we pulled up in front of the center she told me I had tricked her, and that she was not going to that job. I told her she had to and she told me that she hoped that she would fall on the tree roots and break both of her legs and I would have to call 911 and then she couldn't go to work. I almost drug her inside and once we got indoors, she was her pleasant self but she was mad at me and I could tell! I had been telling people for years to just take people to day care or senior centers, have them go as volunteers if they were too high functioning as a participant but to take them and the center would take it from there. I had once again not followed my own advice and it made her adjustment more difficult. She also continued to complain all the way there every morning. She would even tell waiters in a restaurant that I had put her to work as a (she would turn to me and ask for the word) volunteer, and then tell them that meant I made her go to work every morning and she didn't even get paid!

Pain or Privilege?

There was a lot of pain at this time and boy was that "all about me". My lifestyle had changed for I had someone at home for whom I was responsible, which meant it could not be "all about me." Mom also had changed her entire life and all she wanted was a little attention and I just didn't have it to give with the way things were arranged. I was having a difficult time but I hadn't really thought about the changes or planned for them, I just whined to myself. However, this was my mother and she could read my feelings so she picked up on my unhappiness—no wonder she wanted to go home to her house! Change, even when it is for the best is difficult and requires adjustment. We had to adjust! I also realized when she couldn't stay alone any longer but I should have noticed when she appeared so distraught and clearly not have waited until 'she told me'. Do you see how I continued through this entire process to allow her to be the mother, and totally forgot all the things I knew professionally? I would have spotted the signs immediately had it not been that she was my mother and an impact on my life. I rationalized that I could not leave her alone all day, but it was o.k. to take her to a program from 9:00 A.M. to 3:00 P.M. Then leave her at home from 3:00 P.M. until whatever time I could get home. I guess there was just a moratorium on any problems from 3:00 P.M. until 6:00 P.M. in my mind! I asked her to interview for a job with no option to say no. If she had no option then it needed to be presented in that manner, I knew it but I did not do it! I did not follow my own advice and for that there was pain. She was angry, she let me know it, and that made me feel sorry for myself, which increased my stress, and of course hers too.

In retrospect, and especially since I don't have her with me any longer I realize the privilege of being able to have her at my house. We truly had a wonderful time the majority of the time; when I did not feel like cooking, we went out to eat and the companionship was so pleasant. When friends called, they always welcomed her to join us and they truly enjoyed her company. Everyone repeatedly told me how lucky I was to have such a sweet, kind, friendly mother and I did know they were right. I was really blessed and even with the whining and internal strife, I will always treasure those years. I do wish, also in retrospect, that I could have handled them with more gratitude at the time but I can't change history—and neither can you! Be happy for what was and let go of what could have been.

If you are just starting on this journey, plan for it; if you need alone time, then work it into the end of your day. It is possible to find someone to provide transportation to and from a day center that is open during regular working hours. Had I arranged for Mom to attend a center like that or to go to one of the homes where I worked, instead of taking her home, to be alone and unsafe, I still could have had my 'unwind' time and we both would have been less stressed and enjoyed our time more. However, I was too proud to ask for assistance or to even take advantage of the options that were already available to me. I could have hired someone to come in for a few hours at the end of the day and fix dinner. Imagine, coming home to a safe content mother and a delicious healthy dinner on the table. There are creative ways to solve difficult issues that are truly win-win and especially when we are caregivers, we need to look for them.

3

Never Forget
Always Remember

ever Forget: Never forget what they did for you and what is really important about a person. If you can, look for their external and internal beauty, hold their hand, hug them, and share a treat, music, or something you always enjoyed together. Concentrate on what is still there not on what is missing. They may not be the person they used to be but they are still as important.

Always Remember: What they did for you, how it felt, the important times together. Share the fun of the long past, which they will remember best. Think back to what you remember and certainly, it will not have anything to do with their 'great conversation' or 'intellect' it will have to do with what made you smile, laugh, cry. Those are the things to look for now and there is a lot to enjoy, but you may have to search.

Now What Does That Mean?

When we get caught up in the stresses of everyday life and especially when it is complicated with illness it becomes very easy to concentrate on the things that aren't really important. Never forget why you care about each other and always remember what is important. If you get caught up in the difficulty of everyday tasks or "making a point" your quality of life will decline rapidly. It is essential that you never forget that the person for whom you are caring, needs for you to be alive and healthy to "be there" for them as the disease "takes away their capacity". If you insist on doing everything for them for 24/7 you will burn out, become ill, perhaps even die and then they will have no one—the caregiver must take care of themselves first. Think of it like the instructions on the airlines, "First put the oxygen mask on yourself and then on the person for whom you are responsible."

One of the first things you will have to change is the way you interact; enjoy the ability to converse with your loved one and do not worry about the conversation. Here is an example of what I am talking about. I have been a professional working with Caregivers, primarily those caring for someone with Alzheimer's disease, for over a decade. Caregivers are always reluctant to seek help or even to attend support groups. They often say things like, "It is my Mom that has the disease; it shouldn't be about me." I explain that their life changes as a caregiver and they need to take care of themselves. Now that I am in the role of the caregiver, this feeling they are expressing is becoming clearer to me. It truly seems selfish and almost like whining to discuss the emotional turmoil around caregiving. Caregivers by nature are concerned about others so it is especially difficult when "you feel like you are going crazy" and very guilt provoking to have to deal with those feelings when you are truly so concerned about your loved one. I hope sharing my story will help others identify with their feelings.

Our story—from my perspective!

It was a beautiful Fall day, Sunday, just perfect for a walk, a day to go to breakfast, and relax. Mom and I were together at my house and ready to have a lovely day; I was rested and had no specific pressures it was a day to enjoy. When I went to take the dog out for a walk I told Mom we would go out for breakfast when I returned. When I got back she wasn't dressed but she was very proud, she had made up the bed and put the evening dishes in the dishwasher. I was pleased because she felt like she was making a contribution and I made a mental note that I needed to give her more things to do because feeling useful is so important to all humans. I was very calm and printed some things on the computer, and washed the dog bowls while she got dressed. It took a long time for her to dress but we weren't in a hurry. She decided that she wanted to pay for breakfast and we got out her traveler's checks but couldn't find her driver's license. I asked her why she didn't put it in the same place in her purse every time so it would be easy to find and she said she did. We found it in a different place in her purse and she didn't know how it had gotten there. We didn't talk much as we walked to the restaurant and I even teased her about being "Pa Kettle" because if I slowed down so did she and she continued to walk about 4 steps behind me. I told her how far we still had to go and I watched to be sure she wasn't getting winded. She was very concerned about where we were going and if she had been there before. I assured her she had and tried to recount times we had gone there and with whom. When we finally got to the restaurant, she did think she had remembered being there before. As usual when I asked her what she planned to order she asked what I was having and said she would have that too. I was a little smarter this morning and showed her something on the menu that I knew she would like and it was $1 cheaper than what I was getting so she was especially pleased. I love to read the paper on Sunday morning and I gave her the parts of the paper she liked. She just wanted to watch the people. I decided to read anyway and she truly didn't seem to mind though she doesn't like me to read. Our breakfast came and she was just delighted with hers and actually ate it all. We've been discussing eating as she has been losing weight and has really decreased her portions. We had such a pleasant time and I did not mind not finishing my paper. We walked back and talked about the flowers in bloom. It was very interesting as she interpreted what she saw as we walked along. There was a truck sitting at a curb and someone taking some equipment out of a restaurant. She said, "Look over there, those people's stuff is on the street and someone is hauling it away." I started to explain what I thought was happening and then realized that it didn't matter. Either of our interpretations were o.k.; she could be right and I could let it go, it is a matter of dignity. I knew this intellectually but I just needed to practice. So often, I had been correcting what she said and she would tell me, "I'm just making conversation, don't get mad at me." I think I had been paying more attention to what she was saying because I had been assessing her and she obviously, had felt that scrutiny and responded to it appropriately. When we got home, she was very pleased that we had had such a nice time and so was I. But there is a part of me that felt like it was work rather than just enjoying time together. Things had changed between us and I was feeling and struggling with the change. It was very hard to determine if my changes were making her more dependent or if I was in denial about her capabilities and looking for excuses.

Now that was the story when I was at my best, early in the day. I handled everything so well it could have even been titled, "The normal day in the life of a caregiver," though I felt it to be challenging. Now I will tell you what I will always refer to as "The Sweater Incident," a story that will resonate with those of you who absolutely find yourself at the end of your rope on a regular basis. This is 'all about you' and you need to know that this is the sign that you are doing too much and it isn't good for you but it isn't good for them either!! Yes, I am preaching!

Every evening, right before bed we took the dog out for his nighttime walk. Now, I really wanted to do this quickly and by myself. However, it was dark and my Mom thought I should not go out alone. That subject usually would make me bristle a bit because I truly felt I was better off alone if we had a problem. However, she was my mother and she was meant to protect me! I once told her that I would be safe with a dog the size of our dog and she said, "Well, what if they shoot him?" Fortunately, the retort is that they would shoot us too or who were "they" anyway flitted through my mind but only briefly and I never said it out loud. So it was a foregone conclusion that we would walk the dog. When we got ready to go out the door, Mom would go to the bathroom and she wasn't fast with that little procedure and then I would go to look for her and she would be in the closet. Of course the dog was not waiting patiently either. I would ask her what she needed and she would come out all pleased with herself because she had her big wool sweater on and she had my sweater too. Now we lived in New Orleans and there were very few evenings when one could tolerate a sweater and often when it was 90+ degrees a sweater was truly uncomfortable. So she would hand me the sweater and 6 out of 7 times I would just say thanks and off we would go. However, about once a week I would just lose it!!! I would say, "Mom, I don't need a sweater, it is like going from the refrigerator to an oven and you want me to wear a sweater!" She would look at me so sad and stricken and say "Don't get mad at me you need your sweater!" The look would bring me to my senses and I would obediently and guiltily take the sweater and either put it on or put it on the inside doorknob as we would go out the door. Now why was that sweater such a problem for me? I would feel so terrible and I truly couldn't understand why I would just have to have this meltdown. In addition, when I didn't have the meltdown I would feel my entire body tense and I feel certain that my blood pressure was rising. It is no wonder that after we got back from walking the dog I treated us to a large dish of ice cream (it's my story and I am sticking to it) and if Mom didn't want all of hers I ate that too. It will come as no surprise that I gained 60 lbs in 2 years, which was yet another sign that I was not taking care of myself, certainly not the wisest choice for me or for Mom.

Pain or Privilege?

What I hope that I am sharing with others are examples of practicing new skills and sharing feelings, not whining. I am feeling loss and it is hard to define. I don't know if it is losing an old way of life, shifting roles, or not being able to be myself with the one person who always accepted me unconditionally. She needs my unconditional acceptance now and I don't know if I want to "mother" my mother. I know she deserves it and I am the one doing it but I just feel so sad because I am losing something I need. That is all about me, and that is just what feelings are, they are about us. It is stressful to address this but it is so necessary when one is placed in the caregiver role, even if the role is premature.

It is so easy to feel guilty when I have expressed negative emotions in relation to caring for my mother. I truly know it is a privilege to be able to care for her. My approach to all challenges has always been to find a new way of looking at things. I am determined to find new ways of perceiving the changing relationship with my Mom. The first step is to remind myself how lucky I am that I still have my mother and I am in my fifties. Most important of all she is living and I can hug her and hugs are more important than anything else is.

The role that your loved one has held in your life is going to change early on and continue to change. This person can no longer be the parent, spouse, sibling or friend and confidant as they once were. You are now going to have to find a way to accept that they are here but in a different role. Initially, it is very difficult for both of you as they slip back and forth in and out of the role as they have "good days" and "bad days". It gets easier for them as the disease progresses as they are less aware of how much the role has changed. Unfortunately, it becomes more difficult for the caregivers as they are aware of the loss. Both of you are going through tremendous change and loss and that requires that you go through a grieving process. It is essential that you both get into support groups, which should be available for both of you through your local Alzheimer's Association; there are also caregiver support groups with other Alzheimer's organizations such as the Alzheimer's Foundation and with hospitals and in Area Agencies on Aging.

You need to learn to ask yourself, "How important is this issue anyway and what is it really about?" I was too tired at the end of the day and I had made no provisions for taking care of myself. I should have taken an evening off a week and had someone come to stay with Mom so I could do something for myself. I actually had someone come to stay with Mom one night when I had a meeting, and I was so worried that she would be offended. When the woman arrived Mom said, "How nice you came to visit us!" I said, "I ordered pizza and the two of you are going to have a great time," as I headed out the door. Mom said, "Don't you want to eat pizza with us?" I grudgingly said "No, I am going out to dinner." She just hugged me and said, "Have a good time." Now, isn't that a lot easier than yelling at my Mom, feeling guilty, and eating ice cream for comfort? In addition, it provided her with someone else to enjoy, imagine that he or she can get as tired of us as we get of them. I have rarely ever heard a caregiver mention that issue but as a professional, I always point it out, as it was really true. However, my professional judgment continued to be clouded as I only had someone come in to stay with Mom if I had a meeting to go to, I never once did it for her and my pleasure. In retrospect, I realize that had I not played the role of the martyr (even subconsciously) and had arranged to continue to "have a life" separate from my mother, we would have been able to manage much longer than we did. By not taking care of myself, ultimately, I put our time together at risk. While I cannot change history I can make myself vulnerable and share this story with you. I hope that if you are new at this care giving business you can learn from my mistakes and restructure what you are doing and you can change that today. It will be life altering for both of you and it will clearly enhance your quality of life.

4

Never Walk Alone
Always Accept Help

<u>ever Walk Alone:</u> It is critical that every caregiver understand, he or she cannot do this alone. It does not matter if you think there is no one else to help you. If you try to do this without assistance you will burn out very quickly, you will become ill, and you could even die. This is the most serious thing for you to understand, it is essential for survival.

<u>Always Accept Help:</u> It is very difficult to ask for assistance. Often, family members offer only criticism, friends say they wish they could help. For a variety of reasons, most caregivers refuse assistance when it is offered. You not only must accept help you need to plan for it and the earlier the better.

Now What Does That Mean?

The first sign that you are truly a burnt out caregiver is when you think you are the only one that can take care of your loved one. Now, some of you started out that way, so how could you possibly be burnt out? Maybe the point should be, even if you do not want to be away from them, they have the right to be away from you. You need to think of doing things "for them" not "to them".

Caregivers provide many objections to accepting help, some are as follows:

It is just easier to do it myself!

They only want to be with me, when I am out of their sight, they become frantic!

I am the only one in my family or I am the only one in my family who has time!

They are not ready for day care yet!

It really is not that bad!

No matter what anyone suggests, you have a reason why not to take the advice:

We do not have the money for that!

There is no one that can really help!

No one wants to help!

I made a vow "in sickness, and in health"!

Why would I go to a support group, I am not the one with the illness!

However, you do not really understand!

I am getting enough sleep!

I think I can do this for a while longer!

Right now, we are o.k!

I am afraid others will find out how bad it really is!

What if other people do not understand and they make fun!

What if they are not kind to my loved one—he/she can be difficult!

It is imperative that you understand from the day of the diagnosis that you cannot do this alone. While it is truly a privilege to be the primary caregiver and accepting that privilege is admirable, it is so important that you think about them and think about their quality of life. Do not measure quality of life by how many hours you spend together, measure it by how enjoyable the day was today. All relationships have struggles and that is necessary, however if someone is so ill with cancer that they are in a persistent state of agitation or pain, you do something about it. Brain Degeneration (regardless of the cause, Alzheimer's, Vascular, or other disease process) needs to have the same level of analysis—do not think that this is "just the way it is"; there is much you can do to enhance the quality of life and it isn't in a medication bottle. First, it requires you to truly understand and accept that this is a devastating disease and your loved one is only going to get worse and second, like any other disease process it is going to require drastic change.

Let us compare the symptoms of Dementia (regardless of what causes the symptoms) to other disease for a few minutes to assist with the rethinking process. When my dad got cancer, the treatment drastically changed his life. In 1979, he was diagnosed with prostate cancer and then the surgeons did drastic surgery with no reconstruction or pills available. He was only 59 years old, which to me at age 30 seemed really old, now at my age I realize how young it was! The surgery, removing the prostate, changed the way he went to the bathroom and made him sexually dysfunctional. While it was not fair, and it was surely kept private, it totally changed everything he did and must have had a profound effect on my mother who was only 57. He even had to change the style of clothing he wore because he wore a leg bag and would have been so embarrassed if it showed. I am sure they changed the amount of time they could attend functions and even many of his work habits. If you think about it, probably even in the men's room, for him, things changed. However, even as we discuss it here, we take it in stride and totally accept the fact that all of this was inevitable with cancer and was necessary for him to be able to be alive and functioning on a daily basis. I feel sure his siblings probably did not even know what the surgery entailed. His children clearly did not think about the changes and we deemed him too old for it to matter anyway. As usual, for the spouse it must have been the most difficult and for the relationship, much had changed. Was it fair, of course not, but it was accepted and life moved on.

He had another illness, Guillain-Barre' Syndrome, which was originally diagnosed and they just accidentally found the prostate cancer while testing and treating the disease. He was very able to fight and recover from that disease though he had been told that he would probably never walk again. However, he was tough, independent, and in control of his life, even though he had a lot of difficulty dealing with being ill for the first time in his life. In 1981, he lost the job with the company for whom he had worked since 1955 and he also chose to move back to his hometown as he felt like Mom would be better there without him. I do remember my Mom being very opposed to leaving her really nice house in Denver and moving back to their rental home in Sterling but dad was in charge. However, at the time they moved he was very ill again and I truly think he thought he would not survive. My brothers and brother-in-law actually made the move and they threw away at least 50% of dad's stuff. It was necessary, because the home they were moving to was only half the size of the one they had but I do not think anyone felt particularly guilty about the move or the loss of the junk. My dad collected everything because he was "going to use it someday." He actually could turn junk, especially wood, into treasure but he was probably not going to be able to do any of that again and amazingly, he never seemed to miss all of the stuff that was gone.

Dad was tough and determined and though life had changed drastically, he and Mom persevered and though he had several other bouts with illness, primarily from the cancer, they changed their lives and had some quality of life during those years. I do remember my Mom being very unhappy the first couple of years but she had an almost magic ability to adjust and accept whatever happened in life and she still showed much more happiness than unhappiness. For the majority of the next ten years they were functional and happy, Mom retired early at age 62 but dad refused to retire and even went back to the company for whom he had worked all those years, though they now had beat him out of his retirement because of the work interruption.

In 1990, (at age 70), my dad seemed to be slowing down. He officially retired from his primary job and then took on a job assisting an old friend and competitor in running his business. When this friend died, dad took on the task of helping the family close out the business. Because he was so indebted to this work, he apparently neglected his own health and by the spring of 1991, it could no longer be neglected. By then, his cancer had advanced and he had 17 bone tumors and 2 in his lungs. This was the beginning of a very difficult bout with the end of life decisions. He and Mom had never planned for end of life, truly never discussed end of life except for some funeral arrangements they had made much earlier and then cancelled, probably due to lack of payment in the years when dad had been so ill. Not unlike many people in that generation, they kept all matters of finance and end of life very personal. I tried to make decisions for dad, primarily because I was available and because I knew the long-term care field. However, my Mom did not trust the two of us together, especially near the end of his life, and would not let us discuss "end of life care." In those last two years dad made many decisions I did not agree with. One of them was his insisting on getting into the car, after the hospitalization and driving the 130 miles home to Sterling. I knew he should not be driving and I was concerned for Mom's safety riding with him. However, though physically ill, my dad was in charge and he was capable of making decisions, though not necessarily wise.

There are several reasons for me telling about my dad in this book. One is because there is a parallel in illness. It truly seems like all of us when dealing with brain degeneration illness we tend to refuse to accept it as an illness and thus refuse to make the necessary though difficult changes based on this illness. We also refuse to plan for the inevitable, which is usually not the case with any other physical illness. In addition, when we are wrestling with what is best for the ill person, it is important to determine whether they are truly capable of making decisions, though sometimes unwise. If it is a physical illness that does not primarily affect the brain, then some can still think clearly and make decisions. Someone who has a degenerating brain cannot make decisions consistently about safety and cannot be left alone—regardless of their wishes. I just want to be clear that you understand while I did not agree with many of my dad's decisions, they were his decisions. My mother's illness is very different; I could not allow her to make decisions for she is truly incapable of making them due to her disease. Letting her decide would become neglect and even abuse on my part. There were times with my dad's illness that I truly disagreed with his decisions for they were not wise but he was capable of making those decisions. I would equate that with each of us choosing, to not exercise, to eat too much, to eat unhealthy things, even to smoke. They are not wise choices, we certainly know better but we choose the wrong things anyway. My mother wanting to stay in her own home, where she couldn't remember to eat and didn't know not to give her credit card to strangers or not to let strangers into her home is not the same kind of unwise choices—she had to have the decisions made for her. Though it seemed easier with my mother's "Edith Bunker type personality," it was just as difficult because there was even more guilt when I knew I was not making the choices for her that she would have preferred and that she was virtually defenseless.

It is in this section of the book, though it may appear to be self-serving that I take an excerpt from my first book <u>Alzheimer's Disease: Help and Hope</u>. It is so essential that you understand this disease process before you can even begin to discern whether your loved one can make their own decisions. This information is to assist you with understanding so you can move forward. Do not use this information in place of the complete medical and neurological examination that I discussed in chapter 1 of this book. Only the best geriatric physicians can determine if what your loved one has is treatable, do not rely on guesswork with something so important. When your loved ones have the symptoms of dementia (regardless of the cause) confirmed by a complete examination, then you need to know what it means and what to expect and that is where my "lay" explanation is very useful for you as follows:

It is important, for me, to make you aware that in explaining Alzheimer's disease I am not describing this in medical or scientific terms. I refer to this description in "lay" terms or as some might say, "Explaining in Plain English". Through the years, I have tried to come up with analogies and descriptions with which someone can identify to make this disease more understandable. My premise is that with increasing understanding of the disease, care becomes easier. Questions that I am most often asked and my explanations are as follows:

Alzheimer's disease is a regressive degenerative brain disease:

Because of brain deterioration, the memory (information) is eliminated, in all or part, in the reverse order that it is acquired and stored. A person with Alzheimer's disease may not be able to acquire any new information at all, or they may just acquire bits and pieces. A way that is helpful to understand how this works is to draw a large dark squiggle on the blackboard. Underneath it put dates starting from 1920 on the left and going to 2000 on the right. Now I want you to think of this as the brain of a person with Alzheimer's disease. Take a blackboard eraser and start at the right (2000 side) and erase back towards the 1920 side, do not erase everything all the way, but erase the most on the 2000 side. Now look at the spot (brain) on the blackboard. No matter how good you eraser is, it does not erase every spot uniformly. However, in the part where you erased the hardest, most of the mark is gone.

This is a very simplistic illustration of how regression in the brain of an Alzheimer's person is working. It is almost impossible to determine how the erasing stops but we do know that the 1920 information will be there the longest (regressive-reverse order it was stored). That is why a person with Alzheimer's does not know if they ate breakfast but for them recalling something from second grade is clear. That is why they do not know your name and they are looking for their mother. That is why they are not at home, even if they are living in their home where they have resided for twenty years or they have just been placed in a facility. It is also why they even think their spouse is a stranger, chances are that the spouse has changed over time and they don't look like they did previously. They can and will have a clear or lucid moment, hour or day depending on how efficient the eraser has been; some of those chalk areas remain even in the 1990's or 2000's. That is why it is not delusions nor hallucinations for them to describe things in the 1940's or 1950's as if it were today; in their brain it is actually the 1940's or 1950's or pieces of each. If we can understand and imagine that we are in that time with them, life will be easier for both of us. It is not strange behavior for either of us it is responding to and understanding the needs of someone with a regressive brain disease.

Diagnostic procedure:

Officially, the absolute way to determine if it is Alzheimer's disease is to have a brain biopsy, which is usually done at autopsy. However, there is as much as 90% accuracy in diagnosis by doing a battery of tests to rule out other disease processes. In order to be diagnosed with Alzheimer's disease it is essential to have an extensive exam that includes MRI, PET, etc. This is important to be certain that the person does not have another disease that requires different and specific treatment.

When the Diagnosis is Probable Alzheimer's disease:

This means the individual has memory impairment not complete memory obliteration. This impairment is most significant in the ability to learn new information or to recall previously learned information. In addition, they must have at least one but may have all of the following cognitive disturbances:

Aphasia is a language disturbance that can be divided into two categories, expressive and receptive. Expressive means they cannot say what they want to say. Speech may come out in mixed up words, or the person may be unable to form words at all. Receptive means that they cannot make sense of what you are saying. They may have one, both, or none of these problems and this can change over time depending on how the disease continues to affect their brain.

Apraxia is a problem with carrying out movement despite intact motor functions. My understanding of this is that the brain is giving inaccurate signals to the rest of the body and consequently things do not work right. This may result in changes in movement of the body and can be an explanation for why a person with Alzheimer's paces. It is as if the body does not know how to stop, though other 'schools of thought' are that pacing is a sign of boredom. It also might explain involuntary movements, stops, starts, shuffles, small steps, rigidity, inability to use eating utensils, etc. Motor dysfunction creates safety issues and can result in falls and injuries.

Agnosia is an inability to recognize or identify familiar objects. This too can create many problems for functioning in any environment. There are both dignity and safety issues involved. Not being able to differentiate between a telephone and a remote control is embarrassing, describing a table as a plate holder may be amusing (to others), and yet confusing ones toothbrush with the safety razor is dangerous.

Executive Functioning Disturbance, such as planning, organizing, sequencing, abstracting is something that seems to be taken for granted. Each function we perform requires many steps and thought processes. If a person with Alzheimer's disease has disturbance in this area it becomes very difficult to do everyday tasks around the home, and even maintain personal care. It is virtually impossible to carry out more complex tasks like shopping for groceries, cooking a meal, finding your way home, etc.

These things have to be apparent to the degree that they affect their ability to perform in everyday life in order to receive this diagnosis.

Review this criterion and imagine the loss of ability a person with Alzheimer's disease faces. Imagine what it must feel like to not learn, retain new information, express words, understand words, move around safely, identify familiar objects or even keep track of what you are doing and where you are going. In addition, it only gets worse and just because there are not problems in some of these areas today does not mean there will not be problems in those areas soon. Really think about this, think about it for your own life and you will begin to understand and appreciate the person for what they can do and you need to stop concentrating on what they can no longer accomplish. When working with a person with Alzheimer's disease it is essential to keep the magnitude of their disease process in mind, not so you can pity them, but so you can accept them for the person they are today. Then go one step further, form a new type of relationship with this person and enjoy each day with them.

Dementia:

Another subject that seems very confusing is this term called dementia. Many people say that the person with whom they are involved does not have Alzheimer's disease they just have Dementia. Dementia though listed as a diagnosis code for insurance purposes, is not really a diagnosis, it is much better described as a symptom. An easy to understand analogy with dementia is vomiting.

Vomiting is something that is universally known, and with the word comes an actual picture of something with which virtually everyone is familiar. The cause for vomiting can be self inflicted (from too much food or drink), a form of wellness (such as in pregnancy), induced by medical treatment (such as radiation or chemotherapy), psychologically induced (anorexia or bulimia) or an actual result of something that is wrong with the gastrointestinal tract. To be even more specific the different types of vomiting could be discussed (projectile, bile, etc.) but that is not as commonly known. The point is that vomiting evokes a picture of something and the treatment for it is essentially the same regardless of the cause. In addition, regardless of the cause it is accepted as uncontrollable and the person with the symptom is not blamed or mistreated for having it regardless of the mess or inconvenience it creates.

Dementia for all visible and real purposes looks about the same; it is a progressive-regressive pattern that requires the person with it to require assistance with their activities of daily living. The cause for the dementia is the actual diagnosis. Alzheimer's disease is the leading cause of dementia, with vascular (from strokes) as the second most common cause for dementia. There are many other causes for dementia but they are all in very small percentages. Currently, most Dementia's are referred to as Alzheimer's. There are many reasons for this generalization and probably the most common is that when you say Alzheimer's it seems to have become known enough that most people recognize it. If you say dementia or specify such as vascular dementia there tends to be more confusion. The cause of the dementia makes relatively little difference in the treatment. Persons with a degenerating brain, regardless of what is causing the degeneration, need to be accepted as persons with a disease process that is uncontrollable. They need to be treated with the kindness, understanding and positive interventions that minimize the disease process and maximize their quality of life.

Now that you understand, and probably recognize a lot more of the disease process in your own loved one you will realize why you have the privilege and yes the responsibility to make the choices that are best for them. It is also more understandable for you to realize that from the time of diagnosis they need to have something to do with their lives, regardless of how boring it may seem to us, which allows them to have peers and the ability to feel useful and meaningful. Nothing is worse than to just sit around waiting to die or being alone and frightened. We have a responsibility to find environments that are safe and interesting for them. They are available and we can find them and we even can afford them but it takes a change in thinking and some life changes, just as if they had cancer or diabetes—illness creates the need for change in order to effectively deal with the illness.

Our story—from my perspective!

I am stepping back in time to share with you the experience I wrote in my journal the day after I realized that I was actually leaving my Momma home with the dog and knew I could not continue to do this any longer, for I was truly putting her in harms way!

I was so frustrated I could just cry! I would have cried, if it would not have upset my Mom to see me crying. That is just another thing that is so difficult about care giving; one cannot even have a good cry!

I called several home health agencies that provide private duty. I just wanted to get an idea about what they provide, how much it cost and what I could expect. Now, I really had the advantage because I had worked in the long- term care arena so long. I knew the questions to ask but even as a professional I am amazed at how difficult it was to get the answers I needed. It was so frustrating, being the one that is questioned instead of receiving answers to my questions. I felt like I was shopping for a car! I called and asked for the prices and they would not tell me prices. First, they wanted to discuss my mother with me. I knew they were just doing their job, following their script and getting the information to run their business. However, right then I had questions that I just wanted to ask. I did not really care about their business, I was the customer and I knew what I needed to know. I needed to know if I could afford what I wanted. I was perfectly capable of telling them what I wanted and they should have been able to figure it out by listening to my questions not by filling out the blanks on their forms. Boy did it make me want to train some marketers! Besides, if I could think about what they were doing wrong then I could avoid what I had to do! I had to make some decisions not only about my mother but also for my mother because she could not make the decisions. She thought she was just fine and I was the one who decided she needed help but then I just could not get the information.

Well I thought I had enough problems with the last call that wanted to fill out their information form. The next one said I needed to make an appointment to come in to discuss what we needed. Actually, they wanted me to bring my mother, as they needed to assess her. Now wasn't that great, they are going to figure out in an appointment, for which I definitely did not have the time, how my Mom was really doing. Number one, my Mom would never agree to such an appointment and number two, she was so engaging that they would think she was fine and did not need help anyway. I was truly going crazy as none of this was making sense. So, I just told the woman that I do not have time for an appointment; I did not want my Mom to come for an appointment, as it would upset her. I assured her that I could complete any assessment paperwork. Wouldn't you think I could have just made an appointment? No, she was going to have someone call me. I told her, "You know who I am; you already know my Mom and me." Couldn't you just make the appointment; I needed to get on with this right then! I had to make some decisions and when I had the time and the nerve to make the calls was when I needed the attention, not when someone has time to call me back!!! She was just as polite as could be and just TOTALLY ignored everything I had said and just repeated her previous sentence as if I hadn't spoken at all. She would have someone call me back. You know I have never received that call back. All of you marketers out there, make your calls, call back, this is really important to people. Even if they don't return your calls, call them back, call them back, and call them back. This is so important and if you just show you care, call and listen—it is what you need to do. You can listen and fill out your paper; you can listen and find out what the potential patient is like. You can listen, you can help, and we, the caregivers, making the inquiries need help.

Thank heavens for some people in the world that at least will talk to you, even better will listen to you. I finally got a person who knew who I was. I felt like this was so important because everything I had to say, especially about my Mom, made me sound like I was incoherent. At least, if they already knew me and remembered me they would recognize that I was really stressed—they would know that I must have known what I was talking about, hopefully, they would understand and not judge me too harshly. I still cannot believe that I was concerned about these things. I was astounded that at a time like this I was actually concerned about what people thought. I have never cared what people thought about me. I was concerned though, this was my mother and I was admitting that I, the seasoned professional, could not take care of her, I was asking for help. It was so painful to have had to make such an admission; I really needed to be treated with care. JoAnn was just wonderful, she asked many questions and she sounded like she at least understood but she did not give me prices either. Why couldn't I get prices, why were prices such a secret? If their services cost more than I could afford then I needed to know that up front but didn't they know that I know how much their services were worth and how much I had available. Did they not have plans for alternatives for me if they were out of my price range? Did they feel their prices were too high and I would not continue to discuss other options if they charge too much? I needed to know what I was up against and that began with price. At least she told me how it worked and if they had minimum or maximum hour requirements- but people not in the business would not even know enough to ask that question. At least she was nice to me and we agreed that as soon as I contacted the insurance company I would call her back. At least I would know what was available to me and then perhaps we could discuss price! Oh, my gosh! You don't suppose that she thought that I was comparison shopping and using my Mom as an excuse? I bet that is what was going on, no wonder I was having so much trouble. However, didn't these companies know me better than that and if they really thought I was just comparison shopping couldn't they have addressed it in a way that was less stressful for me. I felt so alone and so confused by the lack of immediate information that was available.

I finally got a "real person" on the phone (after waiting 17 minutes) at the long-term care insurance company. It said on the repeated phone message that I could easily go to the website and get the information but of course, that was not true. I had been to the website and I could not get any of the information I needed. They assured me that they would only pay for Mom to go to day care or have home care not both and the maximum was $50 per day. They would pay up to $100/day for 24-hour care in a nursing home or an assisted living place. What on earth was I thinking when I helped Mom buy this policy. Surely, I had imagined that we would need more help at home and I knew I wasn't going to "put" her anywhere anyway. Well maybe I was just looking at what would be best for Mom at the time. Even if I thought, it wasn't best for her to live at home, I wasn't considering what she wanted or was I? It is so frustrating to think you had planned and now it just was not what you wanted or thought you wanted. Man, I just did not know what I wanted. No that was not true I did know! I wanted my Mom to be well, happy, and self sufficient and able to take care of herself all of her life. I did not apply for the job of being my mother's keeper and it was not because I did not want to do it, I just did not know the right thing to do! It just did not seem right to have to make the changes in her life that are best for her. I just wished she could make these decisions or she would make the decisions that are best for her. Why didn't she just make them a long time ago when it wasn't so difficult?

I sounded like I was "losing it" and that was right, I was. I had to leave my mother at the house that day when I went to work and she should not be left alone. I was not sure what to do, but putting her in harms way, leaving her alone, was definitely not the plan that was best for her. The key here is that I knew what was best but I just could not do it—which, like everything else I was dealing with then was about me, not about her.

If marketers want to be "truly awesome," they need a script that addresses our greatest fears: the fear that maybe our loved ones disease hasn't progressed as much as we think it has, the fear that we will make the wrong decision and feel guilty the rest of our life, the fear that our loved one will hate us for what we have done, the decision we have made, and the fear that friends, family, and neighbors will judge us harshly.

According to the information I had finally gathered I could only afford to place her in 24-hour care. I could not get anyone to stay with her or help me get her ready to go to day care and get day care paid for too. If she did not go to day care, it would cost even more. There is no way that I could get someone to stay with her for $50/day, that was not even minimum wage. I guess the good news was the decision had been made but that was the bad news too; the decision was made based on affordability so I had no choice. I had to move forward, I had to place my Mom in 24-hour care.

I never bothered to call anyone back about what I was doing and you know I was never called back either. Actually, I did put a call in to the owner whose staff person kept insisting that I had to come in for an appointment with my Mom. I told her how frustrating it was for me as a customer who knew what was going on and did she realize how hard it was to get in the door? She said she was sorry, was very polite and did listen. However, she felt certain that the way they were doing things was the right way so I regret having made the call. On top of everything else, I had probably made an enemy from a business standpoint—why don't people realize what is on the other side. Isn't it their business to know, don't they need to know their market? I would be willing to bet, even if they, as a company are doing well. If they would change the script, address the real issues; answer the real questions they could do even better. They could make the difference.

For me, there was really no decision as I already ran the homes where I put my Mom. However, if I had to make the calls to the Assisted Living places and Nursing Homes I now knew the scripts there needed to be changed too! Why on earth hadn't someone figured out what was really going on here?

Pain or Privilege?

When dad became ill, he initially concentrated on getting better and fighting the disease. However, once he had gathered all the information he made choices, for both he and Mom. His focus was to provide for Mom in the event that his illness left him incapacitated or if he should die. The decisions weren't fun, they would not have been the same decisions they would have made had he not been ill. With all serious illness changes have to be made to adjust for that illness and the long-term effect it will have on the persons directly involved.

I continue to repeat that one cannot go back in time; however, if I could I truly believe that I would do things much differently. I will use this part of our story to tell you how it was and then illustrate how it might have been if I would have been capable of following my own advice of, "Never Walking Alone and Always Accepting Help."

When Mom first started having health problems such as the weight problems, her doctor asked her to keep a food diary so they knew what she was eating. She wrote down what she told me she was eating. In reality, if she had been eating what she put on the paper she would not have been losing so much weight. Had I suggested to the doctor (her doctor whom she adored) that we might need to have some cognitive testing done, I feel certain he would have gone along with me. It was early enough that she would have done quite well on the battery of tests; it probably would have shown her inability to truly prepare food and remember to eat that food in a timely manner. There would have been two positive outcomes:

1) it would have been her doctor suggesting that there was a problem, which would have been much more palatable for her and 2)
she could have been given medication that would have held her at
that stage longer. It was only when her doctor told her that since she
did not have weight loss and significant health problems when she
stayed with me but she had them when she was alone that made me
realize something had to change. That was at least a year after the
problems began. She would have been much more able to make the
decision to come and live with me, "Because the doctor said so," and
we could have allowed her more choices about the things she wanted
to bring and she could have participated in the process. Waiting until she could no longer actively participate in the decision making
process, left me making the decisions, feeling guilty and her unable
to make choices that could have been fun earlier. It also could have
prevented the crazy year we had of fighting about everything—in
her words, "I could have been nice to her anyway!" There is no advantage, providing your insurance, financial and legal papers are in
order, in delaying the diagnosis—early detection provides a better
future as in any disease.

Even if we didn't make the earlier diagnosis, I wonder how different our lives might have been if I had figured out a way to follow
my own advice and take care of myself when Mom did need to move
in with me. What if I had enrolled her in a senior program earlier? In
addition, what if I would have arranged for someone to pick her up
after the program and stayed with her at our house until after I went
to exercise in the afternoon. Her long- term care insurance would
have paid for a few hours a day and I would have maintained my
health and well-being. I could have happily shared the advantages

of having my mother live with me that enabled us to both continue our active lifestyles and share quality time together. Had we done it initially, there wouldn't have been all the changing and struggling. I wouldn't have been stressed to the max, gained all that weight and felt so "out of control". The "sweater incident" wouldn't have existed and I certainly would never have been in a position to leave her home with the dog.

Pain or Privilege was a choice I had and it could have been very different if I could have planned for assistance, taken that assistance, and taken care of myself. I am so fortunate that nothing catastrophic happened to either one of us during those few years. Learn from my mistakes; think clearly about all the options available!

However, I waited until Mom was too ill to stay at the senior center. She was not safe staying at home, I was so burned-out that I truly couldn't take care of her any longer and now I was going to have to place her in 24-hour care. I ran 24-hour care, it was excellent care, I believed in 24-hour care but I was in no shape to make decisions. I had waited until our situation got to a crisis situation to make a decision—I had done exactly what I always advised families to avoid. Worst of all I had been leaving Momma home with the dog for a long time.

5

Never Stop
Always Progress

ever Stop: Burned-out, exhausted, and determined to "Hang on, No Matter what"! Paralyzed! When a caregiver reaches this stage, they are in no position to make decisions and they certainly are not capable of making decisions. However, this is the time when decisions are forced and unfortunately, for the caregiver, where the negative statistics are derived. If you get to this stage, you need to get out and it will always be better if you can do it without a crisis for you.

Always Progress: Move forward, which means that finally there is no choice. If you do not move forward for you, then you are unlikely to be around when your loved one needs you. What every person with dementia needs most from their primary caregiver is for the primary caregiver to survive. This is a critical message; it needs to be impressed on caregivers from the first date of diagnosis.

Now What Does That Mean?

Statistically, the caregiver often contracts a major illness and sometimes even dies before the person with dementia, for whom they are caring. Stress, negative lifestyle impact and poor self-care seem to be the culprits creating this significance. Most caregivers dive-in to the caregiver role unaware, totally, of what can and will happen. This is the reason that the Alzheimer's Association has support groups for Caregivers. However, though a support group is essential, understanding the necessary steps for effective care giving is even more essential. The support group tells and shows you what to expect. However, most people become certain that they will not become burned-out. It is that old, "It can't/won't happen to me," syndrome. I know because as the support group leader of many years I still thought I was immune to the "human condition." This premise is not a new or original thought. It certainly dates back to scriptural times—"Love your neighbor as yourself" or if you are more comfortable with the Golden Rule, "Do unto others as you would have them do unto you." It is certainly true for all relationships including marriage and parenting. If you do not take care of yourself, ultimately, you will not be healthy or be effective in continuing to take care of the person for whom you are responsible. So, why is it so hard to take care of ourselves, and why do we wait until it is too late or almost too late? In retrospect, I knew the answer but during the crisis with my mother, you would have thought that I had never had a day of training and certainly had never been in a position to give advice.

So what are these steps? It might be useful to discuss some common illness analogies. If you get a diagnosis of diabetes there is nutritional counseling both for the person who has diabetes and certainly for the person who does the shopping and prepares the meals. Now, if you were to decide that this additional education, more shopping, and new way of cooking are just not fair, it is difficult, it is a lot of extra work and you will not make the changes—what will happen? The person with diabetes will get worse and can even die. Society has very little tolerance for such blatant disregard of following common sense practice of adapting your lifestyle in a way that protects an ill person. Suppose, you find a lump, you have a sore that does not heal, or you experience continuous pain. I think you would agree get to the doctor as soon as possible, because this could be very serious; it could be cancer. If it is cancer, all options will be explored to get the treatment deemed best for your situation. If there is no insurance or if insurance does not cover the best route of treatment, then alternatives, maybe even as unusual as fund-raising are investigated. It is difficult, unfair and certainly requires life-altering changes, but it is embraced and the changes are made. However, when the symptoms of dementia appear, it is hidden, overlooked, and if a diagnosis is made it is then hidden. Then one or two people make unwise choices and just seem to sit around and wait hopelessly for the person to die. Often, the caregiver dies first. It has clearly been defined as "the long goodbye," even by a former President of the United States, and yet the majority of people and health care institutions provide little training or care. The organizations raise money for research, form support groups, and create literature to assist. All of this is helpful but only if the caregiver takes the initiative. The medical people shake their heads, agree something needs to change but within the century they have known about dementia authorities have moved very slowly to create any change in the approach to this disease. Why are there no next steps developed? If a person comes into an emergency room with diabetes, they are monitored so they do not go into a diabetic coma. If they come in with cardiac or stroke symptoms, there is a triage system to make certain they receive immediate care. However, if someone with a dementia comes into the emergency room he or she is usually separated from the person who can answer questions on their behalf. Ultimately, after a catastrophic reaction has been created, they are then strapped to a gurney, given some mind-altering drug and then the person who accompanied them is called in. If, and when, someone is sent home there is no prescription for what should be done and they are on their own to try to prepare for a long devastating life. The person with the dementia is viewed as some sad pathetic person and the majority of their friends and family members just walk away—hoping nothing like that will happen to them. The primary caregivers, even when they are burned-out are criticized for not having done something sooner, or for the decision they have just made, or both. It is as if this illness is the fault of the person with it and the one most directly dealing with that person.

I am of the opinion that when a person becomes the primary caregiver for a person with Dementia, the caregiver must immediately see the doctor and be monitored carefully. They need a prescription that requires them to take care of themselves better than ever before. It is as critical as if they had been diagnosed with diabetes or heart disease, statistically they are at as high or even higher risk for serious illness. Friends and relatives need to be involved in seeing that they have the support they need to make these changes. If as a lifelong friend or family member you are reluctant to go to coffee or lunch with the person with Alzheimer's on a weekly basis—how on earth do you expect their caregiver to do 24 hours a day, 7 days a week, and 365 days a year? If as a lifelong friend or family member, you are unwilling to volunteer to stay with the person so their caregiver can go to dinner or a movie how can you criticize them for becoming burned-out? I know that I went to my physician after my Mother had been living with me for a year. I went for something like sores in my mouth and she could only focus on the fact that I had gained 30 lbs in a year and I must have diabetes. I told her I knew I did not have diabetes that I was taking care of my mother now, I had stopped working out and I ate ice cream every night. She gave me a 1200-calorie diet sheet and ordered a test for diabetes. I just skipped my annual physical that year (only time I have done that since I was 25) because I did not want to discuss my weight with her. In retrospect, I just cannot believe that she did not ask me about depression, ask why my mother was living with me, or ask about anything that should have been a clue that I would have impending health problems. I also have no idea why I did not discuss any of those things with her either. My mother's Geriatrician was a friend of mine. We discussed that she had lost weight and I had gained weight (I even remember joking about I must have found her lost weight) but she did not once ask me how I was doing. In fact, she was very reluctant to order the tests for my mother to have a dementia work-up—though it had been established that she was living with me because she could no longer live alone.

We are not going to change society in time for anyone who now receives a dementia diagnosis. However, we can change our lives in a way that will provide a positive approach to this disease process for both the caregiver and the one for whom they are providing the care.

Our story—from my perspective!

I am going to have to place my Mom in 24-hour care. Now I am very lucky because it is a home for which I am actually in charge. I will have as much control as is possible. So why don't I feel lucky? This is the hardest thing I have ever done. Until now, I thought the hardest thing I had ever done was taking my dad to a nursing home even though he was the one who made that decision. Let me digress.

I had made plans to take dad home with me; I even had the people lined up to care for him at home. After all, I worked in a nursing home; I was in the business of taking care of people so certainly I could take care of my own dad. However, my landlady had other plans; she evicted me because I had only signed a lease for me, not for my Mom (who had been there for three months and now my dad who would be coming there with round the clock workers).

Dad said it was a good deal that he was not coming to my home because he did not want to stay in Denver anyway, he wanted to go home. We tried a weekend in his home and we both realized that he just needed too much help and there was no way Mom could take care of him. It was going to have to be a nursing home. His 94-year-old mother lived in one of the two nursing homes in town, but they did not have a vacancy. My sister, who lived in that town, arranged for him to be admitted to the other nursing home in town.

Care planning said they could arrange for an ambulance to drive him there, for it was 130 miles. But he said no. He said his daughter, the one sitting right there next to him, could take him in her little red car. The decision was made, though not by me, I would be taking him to a Nursing Home.

It was a cold rainy day in May, 13 years ago! My dad had been in the hospital since March 13. He wasn't doing well at all, in fact he was dying. He had told me he would rather be dead than live like this and he truly wasn't a whiner. He was very ill and had become totally dependent. We loaded him into my little red car and with Mom in the backseat we set out for the trip. Dad truly enjoyed the ride and we got there in good time. I drove up to the home and he said, let's just drive past the house first, so we did, then he wanted to drive out past the Burger King (my brother-in-law owned it), and then he wanted to drive past my sister's house and on and on. We drove around for over an hour, and I did not mind because I did not want to take him to a nursing home—not ever, because I felt that I could take care of him.

We seemed to be out of places to drive to so we pulled up to the front of the nursing home. My sister came running out; she was frantic, worrying about where we had been. This was before cell phones so I could not exactly call her but we were about an hour later than she had expected us—because we were avoiding the inevitable.

I helped get dad into the wheelchair and "I put him in the nursing home".

He died in less than a month. It took a lot of work in an intense grief group for me to come to terms with the fact that I had put him in a home. However, the reason I came to grips with it was that it was clear that it was his decision not mine. Now understand, I do not hate nursing homes, because I worked in one. I just felt that I could do it better and it was my responsibility! It was still a sad day in my memory.

Now back to the current story. I could truly no longer take care of Mom and I couldn't leave her at home with the dog. I had checked out the long term care insurance and it would pay for her care but not at home. There are different choices in these policies but right after dad died, when Mom and I had selected the policy we were not planning for Mom to be cognitively impaired, or maybe we did not know the options. No matter, we could afford for her to have 24 hour care in the homes that I had implemented and still ran.

This decision wasn't made lightly, but it was clear, I was a burnt out caregiver and I had gone way past keeping Mom safely at home. There was no choice from a safety and a financial point. I had a space in the 24-hour community I ran, we could afford it, and it was time. I had all the family support possible, they thought it was way past time. I was the problem. One of the reasons I had dedicated my life to long term care was to make certain care was available that was good, especially for a person with dementia. So why was this so difficult?

That was the question a good friend of mine had asked me. He had become a good friend because his Mom had spent her last years in one of the homes. She had died nearly a year before but he kept in touch. In fact, on Mother's Day that year he had invited Mom and me to his home for a crawfish boil. Mom had had such a wonderful time at their home that day. He just happened to call to check to see how my mother was doing and I told him that I was struggling with the decision to put Mom in one of the homes. He just could not fathom why that was difficult. He said, "It should be a no brainer". However, he hadn't forgotten how difficult the decision to make a change was and was very supportive.

I felt like a sneak and a liar and a miserable failure. I knew this would only be successful if I followed my own advice. I needed to not make this a big deal and if it was too difficult for me then I should have someone else do it. I had been giving advice to persons for twenty years on how to manage the final days and the actual move into a long-term care setting. I already knew what to do, what not to do, what to say, and what not to say. I knew the drill but I just couldn't move forward.

Why did I feel like a sneak? I had been planning this for a weekend I had my sister mail stuff from Mom's home in Colorado to the new address. I had bought furniture, I even had made a picture collage and a scrapbook of all the family pictures, I got up at night after Mom was asleep to make labels for all the people in the pictures. I also packed her things while she was sleeping and put them in the car so I could take them without her seeing. No wonder I felt like a sneak! I was sneaking around doing things behind her back. However, I was doing these things for her. My goal was to make sure everything was ready and comfortable so she could settle in with little stress. That was about her and what I needed to do. The feelings were about me! I wouldn't have felt guilty sneaking around if I was planning a surprise party or something fun. It is all about perception and I knew it - but it didn't matter!

Why did I feel like a liar? In my family, truth was the rule, lying was not an option—even calling someone a liar could get you in more trouble than any other four letter word there was. So imagine, how I felt when I was lying to Mom. Well why was I lying? She kept asking me what was wrong and I kept telling her nothing was wrong. I wanted to just put my head in her lap and cry and cry and tell her that I was doing what was best. I should have done that. My Mom might have had dementia but she could have helped me with yet another life passage. For some reason when we are making these difficult decisions, we hide our feelings. I can't change history, but I do believe that if I would have cried with Mom that week we would have both felt better. When you are crying you do not make sense anyway so she would not have understood what was making me so sad. She would have understood that she could comfort me and I am sure she could have helped me through the most difficult time in my life. In retrospect, I wish I would have held my dad and cried in his lap the day I took him to the nursing home. He made the decision and he made me follow through but I did not cry about it until months after he died. I really wished I would have told him how hard it had been—I think he wanted to know and he was not demented. He could have understood. I cried a lot when I came to terms with it in my grief group but I will always have to wonder if it would have been easier for dad if I cried. If for one last time, on that day, he could have been my dad and I his little girl—it was probably the hardest day in his life, too and he had to be strong. Was it for him to be strong or for me? I will never know but you still have time to find out in your situation.

Now the miserable failure part is irrationality and whining! Had I not created the exact care I would have wanted for myself? Had I not helped Mom buy long-term care insurance, which meant we could afford this very option? I was on the inside track of this particular place where she was going to be admitted; I had designed it, hired and trained the staff and had 24-hour access to all information. Now what could be better than that? It certainly wasn't leaving her home in the care of the dog.

In retrospect, what I am trying to share with you is that we just are not rational when we are making major decisions. Do not expect to feel good about difficult and major life changing events; they are difficult and life changing for all involved.

I got everything ready and planned to move Mom in on Tuesday but I did not actually move her in until Thursday and late in the day, after 5:00 P.M.

I just could not do it. I just could not take her to the place she needed most and I decided that I just could not do it. I had a long talk with my brother. Now he and I had not really lived in close proximity or interacted on a routine basis for years. However, one of the good things about Mom living with me was a renewed relationship with my little brother. He was as worried about me "putting Mom in a home" as I was. He asked me when I was taking her and I told him I didn't think I could do it. He said he knew he couldn't do it and I was truly glad he didn't have to. I do not know what we really talked about those two days, I just remember we talked often and I felt so close to him, it is truly a memory to cherish. My sister kept calling and asking me how it was going and I kept telling her everything was o.k. I think I vacillated back and forth between wanting her to feel as guilty as I was feeling and wanting to protect her. We had always shared Mom and dad's care; she had offered to come and help me and she had sent the stuff we needed. It was a very anxious time for her as well and I doubt I made it any easier for her. Being a "bratty little sister" I didn't feel it was "my job" to make it easier for her. How could I feel sorry for myself if I was concerned about her feelings? Again, in retrospect, it is just so amazing how our family roles kick in like we are all little kids again. It will be interesting to see the difference in our perceptions of that time, if we ever discuss those days.

My staff did not understand why I was procrastinating. They kept getting ready for me to "be there" like with any move in and then I just would not show. They would call me and I would make a lame excuses like: the pictures aren't labeled yet, I don't think she is feeling well, I haven't decided quite what to pack, I don't think I am feeling well, it looks like it might rain, or I think I will just wait until morning.

It was Thursday evening, I had a work function to attend and I either had to take Mom to the house or "leave her home with the dog". Now this wasn't really that difficult as I had started leaving her at one of the houses in the evenings if I had to go somewhere. So, I took her there and they had a place for her at the table and she sat down to eat. I hugged her good-bye and told her I was going to a meeting. When she asked me when I would be back I told her it would be late so maybe she could just spend the night. She said, - "Could I really?" I said, "Sure if you want to". Thankfully, my well-trained staff got me out of the door.

Of course, I called back several times and of course, she was content and happy and went to sleep. It really was that easy!

Pain or Privilege?

First, I just wanted to sleep but it was a week before I slept through the night. I would wake up and jump up and look for Mom and then realize that she was not there and then I would lie awake and wonder about her until I drifted off to sleep. I had an incredible amount of family support, as everyone thought I should have had Mom somewhere besides my home for a long time.

The first two weeks did not seem to be much of an adjustment for Mom, which was consistent with my 8 years experience in placement of persons in the homes I had implemented in New Orleans. In addition, consistent with that same experience the adjustment for me, the family member, was more difficult. The first few days I stopped to see her way too often. Finally, on the third day one of my more adventuresome employees said, "Miss Jo, when are you going to stop this? Your Momma is fine, why aren't you?" I then began to try to figure out how to reestablish my life as it was prior to Mom living with me. Our times together still included our favorite places, going out to dinner with friends on Friday night and out to breakfast at our favorite place on Sunday. Even when I took her back to her new home she would say, "Why are we coming here?" and I would reply, "To see your friends," she would say, "Oh, o.k." The only thing she fussed with me about was that she thought her friends, at her new home, would like to come with us too!

It was truly amazing how well she adjusted and how lost I felt as once again my life had totally changed. However, before I got really used to it, just two weeks later, we had Hurricane Katrina evacuation. Life really changed again, more drastically than I could possibly have anticipated.

6

Never Endure
Always Grieve

ever Endure: So often, a caregiver puts their life on hold and just manages to survive. When caring for a person with Alzheimer's or a related Dementia, this period of survival can last for years. It is very important to understand, that this time is far too stressful to exist, indefinitely, in a state of endurance. Stoicism will result in serious health problems, such as teeth grinding, hypertension, ulcers, migraines and even more life threatening illnesses.

Always Grieve: In our society we are taught not to cry, whenever anyone starts to cry the first thing said is always, "Don't cry." In the caregiver journey, not crying is very difficult and unhealthy. From the beginning, the caregiver is losing the person who was once a very integral part of their life. Initially, the caregiver loses the person in the role (parent, sibling, spouse) which they have held and then they continue to lose them bit by bit as the brain degenerates.

Now What Does That Mean?

It is truly amazing how often, as caregivers, we are totally un-aware of what is required to maintain our own good health. The idea of 'sacrificing' ones own dreams and aspirations because of another's illness is truly ludicrous. It is certainly important to accept the responsibility of assisting them with having their needs met. However, it is contrary to everything we have learned in life for it to be possible to put a life on hold for an undetermined amount of time. Change whether positive or negative is difficult and stressful. Change when imposed, either by self or by necessity, is even more difficult to accept. Yet the majority of caregivers, including me, make very unwise choices and set it up so that caring for someone becomes all-consuming. It is in no way to the benefit of anyone to completely dedicate one's life to another. If you do not take care of yourself, follow the plan for your life, take care of your health and mental well-being you will not be fit to live with and you certainly will not be fit to be a caregiver. One can only feel sorry for the recipient of such care, for they are going to become a burden long before their time. We see this type of blatant self-disregard often in this society, which in my opinion is the most selfish thing one can do. It does not usually start out as intentional, it just sort of happens and often it happens because of lack of information and/or just being too tired to create alternatives. Like any other bad habit, it develops and then is difficult to break and the old adage, "miserable but familiar!" takes over. Therefore, to prevent such a bad habit, "do not do it," do not start the bad habit of not caring for and about yourself.

If it is determined, with a proper medical workup, that an individual can no longer safely live alone, then decisions need to occur and they need to be wise decisions. If a friend or family member is planning to move in with the person who can no longer be alone or if that person moves in with a friend or family member, a plan for respite from each other must be established and adhered to from the beginning. The person, who can no longer live alone, because of Alzheimer's or a related dementia, needs a plan for the effective management of their regressive degenerative brain disease. At the time of diagnosis, when they can effectively be a part of the plan, they need to include having activities on a daily basis that includes physical, emotional, spiritual, and intellectual stimulation. This can be acquired a variety of ways but it must be done immediately. The caregiver needs to have a plan to do exactly the same thing. If the caregiver is still working then that will take care of their intellectual needs. However, they need to have a regular work-out routine, they need to have time with friends, they need time to be alone to reflect and worship, and they need to plan occasional weekends away for complete rest.

This is going to be a difficult and emotional change for everyone just as is any major illness and the change will create much loss for the person with the disease and also for their primary caregiver. It is essential to plan for this loss and it is a good idea to work through it together and in a support group. In the previous chapters, I discussed how I wished I had discussed with my dad about his cancer illness and now I wish I had discussed with my mother about her illness. I appeared stoic with both parents; I tried to be very strong and not make matters worse. In that respect, I believe that I made matters worse. It was their last role as my parent, they could have derived comfort from comforting me in my loss and it certainly would have shown that I cared. Wouldn't you just hate to think that if you were going to lose your life, as you once knew it, no one would appear to be sad or care? Now, I am not suggesting that you have funeral practice, be negative, and cry all the time. However, I am suggesting that you spend time enjoying the things you can do and reminiscing about the things you so appreciated in their lives. My son and I so often talk about my Dad and the things he did that we found amazing and amusing. I so wish we had discussed those things with him when we were visiting in the hospital. Instead, we sat around, trying to act as if everything was o.k. and then going home and trying not to think about how ill he was. I bet Dad would have loved to reminisce, even about the things we thought were amusing.

I have done a better job with my Mom, I think, because of my training in this field, for we did enjoy almost all of our time together. However, I often drove myself crazy, trying to do too much and not taking time to live my life. In addition, I wouldn't let her comfort me when I was feeling so sad, but, that wasn't just when I was her caregiver it had been my entire life with my mother. I was always so independent I never wanted her to comfort me or help me but she always could anyway. She was so adept at "playing the role" of sweet innocence, thus my Edith Bunker analogy. However, that innocence was a ruse, for my benefit. She was and still is a mother and it will show with a lucid moment accompanied by a profound statement that shows she has just "read me" in spite of my thinking I have hidden my true feelings. She still did comfort me in her illness. Which is why some of my "duh" revelations such as the idea that she could have dementia, and the fact that I was actually leaving her home with the dog, was a response to my letting down my defenses and her practical answer, "You aren't leaving me home alone, I have a perfectly good dog here to take care of me!"

For most families, and mine is no exception, for a family of a person with dementia this time is one of extreme pain, conflict, and frustration. Family and friends either ignore the person as it is truly "too painful" to see them that way, or they go to visit and then wish they had not gone because it was "too painful." They state, "That isn't the person I knew." For them I believe, the pain is greater than for family members who are able to find a way to have meaningful visits. For those who handle their grief by not visiting or "duty bound" visits, ultimately, live with an incredible amount of guilt and pain for years, which leads to regret after the person actually dies. It is my hope that this book will assist, in a better way for you to address this illness, so family members do not have to feel so much pain, guilt and remorse.

Grief counseling needs to take place at the beginning of this process. There are some anticipatory grief groups now, which should be a required class for all persons with a family member diagnosed with a dementia. I think it is as important as nutritional counseling for a person with diabetes and for their caregiver. Grieving is work and it is a process and just learning about the process can ease some of the pain. After the death of my father, I wasn't doing very well and a friend of mine who worked for a Hospice insisted that I take the 6 week intensive grief class. In that class we did an exercise in which we wrote a letter to the person who was gone and told them everything we wished we had said to them when they were alive. There is enough material on this subject for another book. Please check the books available on grief. If you aren't a reader, then get them in Audio Book or DVD and listen to them. If the first one doesn't work, get another. You do not have to spend money; the local library is a valuable resource on the subject of grief.

My second recommendation is to write this letter to the person who is now living, and then talk about all those things when you visit. It does not matter if they do not appear to understand, though when it comes to feelings and emotions, you will be pleasantly surprised at how much they will understand and you will go away with a sense of relief instead of a sense of dread. If a particular subject makes both of you sad, then change the subject to happier things. Talk about how much you love them, how much they have always meant to you, how much fun you had, how you understand why they told you no that time, the wonderful vacation you shared, the smell of the apple pie or burning leaves. Relive, discuss, and share those experiences and just talk about them and let them interact with you. Get close, hug, cry, laugh, enjoy the time together because one day soon, you won't have that time any longer—the time is too precious to waste on who they are today—their past and your part in that past and almost all feelings can be shared even if they are in end stages of life and don't respond. You can then just hold their hand and say everything you have ever truly wanted to say and do not be at all surprised if they squeeze your hand or make eye contact or smile.

Our story—from my perspective!

In our family, we do not cry. I do remember that old parenting saying, "If you are going to cry, I will give you something to cry about!" However, that was not true of our family. Now, as I have mentioned before we were like the Bunkers in All in the Family. Perhaps, that explains why we didn't cry, I just can't imagine Archie Bunker "taking to" crying much. Now we did have emotion, it was anger, stomping around, door slamming (though that one got you in big trouble) and the intense loud, droning lectures that just went on for what seemed like hours. It is no wonder that when I am sad or upset I tend to just withdraw. I often have referred to myself as a Turtle for I just pull into my shell and though I am there, no one can really reach me. I have clearly been in this shell of mine for several years and it is truly scary to try to figure out when I will actually feel safe to come out again. I so wish I could just cry and cry and cry but right now with the events of my life the past few years it still just hurts too much to cry. It has been my personal experience that sometimes I have to process for a long time, in my shell, and then when it doesn't hurt so much I can actually cry. Now I know the psychologists could have a real heyday with that theory -but it works for me. I also am very prone to feeling sorry for myself during that time period which is another reason that I am so quiet and withdrawn—I am certain no one wants to have to listen to my "pity party."

Mom and I, well mostly Mom, were doing just fine after she moved into the home in New Orleans. Then just two weeks and two days later, along came Hurricane Katrina and we had to evacuate—never to return. Suddenly, our lives completely changed, again forever. We were on the road for a little over a month as I was responsible for the persons who lived in the group homes I directed and for their evacuation. After everyone from those homes were finally settled, Mom and I went to my son's in Illinois. It was a family decision that Mom move into a small assisted living home near my sisters home in the rural Colorado town near where we had grown up. It was like starting the process all over again, however, this time in addition to my burned out state and my life altering trauma from the evacuation, I was truly giving my Mom up, as she would be in a place where at best I could probably see her monthly. This was even more difficult than the first time. However, I was in such a state of shock due to the effects of Hurricane Katrina that it did not really seem to affect me.

In early October, Mom and I flew to Colorado and then drove to the town where my sister lives. That very afternoon, my sister had already gotten her room ready for her; we took Mom to the home where she now lives. However, she recognized it as a place for old people and she said she didn't know anyone who lived there and she didn't want to visit. As always, I could talk Mom into doing anything so she agreed to go in anyway. When she realized we were going to leave her there she was very angry, she said, "I am not ready for this yet and I won't stay." We visited with her for a short period and then we left her there. When I called back, they said she was just fine, happy and visiting. That was so typical for Mom, she has always made the best of everything. Knowing that should have made me feel better, but it did not. It just made me feel guilty and sad that I had to leave her there. I guess I might have felt better if she had been able to stay angry with me, now that does not make a lot of sense, but I would have understood it better. When I went to see her the next day, she seemed fine except she, of course, was ready to go! I told her I had to go to Chicago and she said she had a suitcase. We had been going to Chicago for several years for my grandson's birthdays and for the holidays so she was ready to go. In fact, my last visit with her hospice social worker, 17 months later, the social worker said whenever they mention Jo she says, she is ready to go when I come to get her.

I am going to share my feelings about several really difficult conversations I have had with my Mom since I have become a long distance caregiver. I am still "working through" this whole process. My reason for sharing illustrates the difficulty of this process regardless of the amount of knowledge or training - this is tough stuff!

I spoke to her in early November 2005, I was calling every day and then for a period, I just could not make those daily calls. I changed to calling at least every other day. I have called my Mom every day, unless she was with me, since my dad died on June 7, 1993. Now it just hurts to talk to her and some days I think I can't stand the hurt! I was in New Orleans for a few days during this particular period and I just could not call her then at all—I think I feared that something would "set me off" and I would just collapse. If that happened, I would not be able to move ahead and if that happened I do not know what would happen—well I just could not let that happen, now could I?? As you can clearly see, consistent with the stages of grief, for any loss, there are times when my thoughts are clearly irrational though understandable.

I do want to record the wonderful conversation I did have with her—it was incredibly painful to me but so "good" that it needs to be recorded. My mother in her innocent wisdom has always taught me so much. As you know, I have often referred to my parents as Archie and Edith from All in the Family TV show. Now, I didn't watch TV much in my life and I only really saw a few episodes but those truly depicted my parents. My dad was grouchy and loudly opinionated but underneath had a heart of gold (soft porous melting gold) and he would do anything for anybody—he truly depicted "only the good die young", (we in the field of aging consider 73 as young). My Mother was like Edith, because she always went along with my dad, no matter what and she always seemed so uncomplicated, sweet, and simple. I always told her she was "dumb like a fox"; it was the socialization standard for women in her era. She still spoke her mind and she still had a tremendous amount of influence; she just seemed uncomplicated. You couldn't have a better mother than mine she was always there for me and she was always sweet, gentle, and kind. Even after she became physically ill, she insisted that the doctor had just told her she was fine and she would live to be 100. Even with the vascular dementia caused by the heart problems and the necessary medications she was easy to get along with and easy to take care of and I know that because I wrote "the book" on how to communicate effectively with the most difficult folks with dementia! One day I called her, I was still calling every day then. She said, "Who is this, is this Jo?" I said, "Yes it is." She said, "Good, now will you come and get me, right now!" I said "Mom, I can't come and get you, besides why do you want me to come and get you, you are home; you are in Sterling where you lived all your life." Now, I know that is exactly what I tell people NOT TO SAY, but I did not care I wanted her to understand that I had done the best I could for her and I just wanted her to be home and happy and to not need me so badly—I needed to feel better! She was neither sweet nor cooperative she said, "Sterling, that is just a name, it is a name of nothing, don't tell me a name, Sterling, it is a name, it is nothing! Now you come and get me right now, you and me and the dog we are something, not nothing like a name, we are something and something is together, now hurry up!"

It just broke my heart. I understood and I knew she understood what is "something" and what is "nothing" and though it fed right into my guilt and made it more difficult for me to "not go get her," I do understand what she and I valued. So how did I make that transition? What a tough one! Intellectually, I knew she had a rare lucid moment which she did not have all the time. The conversations since then are usually just idle chatter and generic questions. "Are you o.k., are you well, and is everything o.k. and she loves to hear my voice though she keeps checking to see if it is really me. Actually, she does not know for sure, and I want her to be checking to see if it is really me on the phone. Sometimes her questioning is even more painful than her wanting us to be together. This loss of someone when they are still a voice on the phone or a frail body to hug is so painful. Yet, I can hug her. There are days, still, 13 years after my dad's death that I would give anything to hug or call my dad, to see his smile or to hold his hand! Therefore, I have the best and the worst and I guess to use my Mom's own words, "That is something!"

I often said, "Just because I wrote the book, doesn't mean I have to read it!" Again, I was referring to "my stuff" as Mom had so appropriately called it! Often, on this journey, I just could not take my own advice because it was so difficult! Let me share one of the worst visits that I have had with my Mom. For nearly a month, I prayed every day that I would be granted another visit because the previous visit ended so horribly. I ended the visit by doing everything just wrong that I have ever said not to do, and it truly gave me nightmares! I had come to visit and my usual pattern is to take her with me to my sister's for the day, so I could spend every possible moment with her. I had kept her at my sisters, with me, all day, and I just did not want to take her back, so I waited until the last minute and did not allow enough time for the transition. We were all going out to dinner, and it is just too difficult for Mom to go out to dinner with a group; also my daughter and I were headed back to Denver and I was going on to Chicago the next day. When I took her back, I was in a hurry as everyone else was waiting. I told her good bye and she wanted to go with me. I told her she couldn't go this time and she insisted that she was going anyway. She followed me to the door but I just closed the door and left. Now I have always recommended that the caregiver stay long enough or get assistance when leaving so the loved one did not feel like they had been left behind. However, I was trying to please everyone, my mother and my family, so I just hurried out—I guess thinking she would not really know in a few minutes anyway. I looked back as I drove past and she was standing at the window waving. I knew she was sad and even mad and she had let that show. I of all people know that wasn't the way to leave her but I just didn't know how to fix it and meet my other demands. The good news is that it reaffirmed that we are both better off, and that I am not trying to leave her on a daily basis anymore. The bad news is that I did not go back and fix it and I felt horrible until the next visit. I am sharing this to illustrate why it is important to make your visits good ones and if you do not feel good then take the time to change that feeling. I really realized it with that visit. I just could not get her sweet little uplifted hand and sense of abandonment out of my mind. I will never try to hurry away from her again, it is too painful. In the meantime, I will have to listen to my own advice! Intellectually, I know she doesn't remember that I left her Saturday evening or that she was mad. In fact, she was just fine—I was not! Once again, it was not as much about her, it was about me and that is the way it has always been. What I have to figure out and do is "FOR HER, NOT FOR ME." That is the most difficult part, not just for me but also for everyone. We have to do what is best for the person who is ill and there is a way to do it and to do it right. I can show everyone that way and I guess I will just get to practice.

There is not a day that goes by when I do not wish that I could go and get my Mom and have her near me so I can see her all the time. Intellectually, I know the best thing for her is to leave her where she is as she has extended her life expectancy because she is in the environment where she is receiving the care she needs to receive and she is happy and content—just like she has always been. For me that does not seem like quality of life, but it never did; however, for Mom, it is enough and it is what she needs! What I have been trying hard to concentrate on instead of having her with me is that I can call her every day (did you notice that I am back to calling her every day again). Even though the phone is somewhat difficult for her, I can hear her voice and I can tell her I love her. In addition, I can see her and I can hug her and enjoy her just as she is and I really do know how to do that. However, when it is time to leave, I need to "follow my own advice" I need to be sure she is comfortable and distracted and then sneak out. She truly won't remember when I was there or that I left. Now that is the hardest way for me and it seems wrong on so many levels. However, we are truly talking about me now and it isn't about me anymore it is about her. She needs to be happy and content and in a secure and predictable environment and I need to support her and do my grief work without my Mom! That is the hardest part of all, that is my loss but I owe her that much and so much more. I need to do this for her now, and I will.

Pain or Privilege?

There is no doubt that I have been experiencing the pain, associated with loss. Once again, it is obvious that I am a lot better at giving advice than I am at taking advice. I am not in an anticipatory grief group, I am not in an Alzheimer's Support Group and I try to ignore my feelings wherever possible. It is no wonder that I have been "stuck" for over a year. My son, keeps saying, "Mom, are you okay, what are you doing, it looks like you are going around in circles?" To which I often agree, "Most of the time, I feel as if I am going around in circles." I do have a choice and for me that choice has been to crawl into my shell and let it turn in circles until I feel I have enough courage to poke my head out and go to the next step.

I think I have finally poked my head out by writing this chapter of my book. I finished this book in August of 2005. However, it was a very different book then with an entirely different set of chapters. Then it was the journey of the caregiver who had run the caregiver race, though overextended and had made it to the finish line and then crashed! However, as with so many finish lines in life, I realized it was just the beginning! As I periodically got enough nerve to poke my head out I rewrote the Ten Absolutes for Caregiver Decision Making, I rewrote the titles of the Chapters and then, one by one I rewrote most of the chapters. I had new lessons to learn about this journey. I had new perspectives to review and the most painful of all was the one of the long distance care giver. Had it not been for Hurricane Katrina, I feel certain that my journey as a caregiver would have been very different. According to Mom's heart doctors, she would have been very lucky to live to the end of 2005. The story and the original book would have ended with my rejuvenation as I "got my life back" and my mother and I sharing wonderful moments for those few remaining months. I would imagine that we would have gone home for Christmas, (I just could not get it that traveling was not in her best interest) and she might have blissfully slipped off to the hereafter after a holiday celebrated with all her family and friends, doesn't it just have that Norman Rockwell feeling? I am such an incurable romantic!

I guess, once again obviously with tongue in cheek, I was blessed for more! Here-in lies the privilege. As I have already shared, my life changed forever. I had so many lessons to learn about life, for me and for my Mom! The best is that with consistent care, my Mom has physically stabilized and her heart seems to be fine. She has had numerous hospitalizations and her brain degeneration has rapidly progressed. She is now on hospice but she not only lived to the end of 2005 she has lived into 2007. Her days are spent in a happy world, surrounded by people who care for her and I can truly say whenever I talk to her she is always pleasant and cheerful. It is truly a privilege to be the daughter of someone with such a wonderful grasp on the true value of life and acceptance. When I talk to her, sometimes she knows me but most of the time she just asks how I am and chats about all the good things in her life and what she had done all day. Often, those things are reliving periods in her life that, for her, must have been the best. Her parents are alive, my dad is alive, and her children are small, so cute, and so content.

Many people remark that it is so sad to see her this way. I too am sad that I don't have a Mom to "tell my troubles to." However, when I can think about her, it isn't sad; she is so happy. In addition, I am truly grateful that I can still hear her voice, tell her I love her and hopefully see and hug her one more time, even spend the day with her and just see her so peaceful and happy. I want to hang on forever, though all the signs are telling me that there is a very short period of time remaining.

My natural inclination is to put my life on hold, go there and spend every moment with her that we still have. However, I would guess, and I am slowly learning, that being with her constantly would totally steal her current happiness. What I need to do is really start taking care of myself, finish this book, cry a lot, and get back to truly helping others on this journey.

There is a great deal of value in having experienced something if one is going to be of assistance to others. Technically, in this journey I know the difference between sympathy and empathy. I have clearly decided that the only part of this journey that I have not experienced is as a spouse. For the first time in my life, I am ready, willing and able to do whatever is necessary to serve in the capacity for which I have received so much talent and experience.

7

Never Explain
Always Act

N ever Explain: Too much information is not good. Keep answers honest, succinct, confident, reasonable and acceptable. Ask yourself, are you explaining to convince yourself or to convince someone else?

Always Act: You have a responsibility to act in the best interest of your loved one for whom you are responsible. Take that responsibility and move forward in their best interest. This is about them, not about you!

Now What Does That Mean?

When I shared the painful mistakes of interacting with my Mom in the past chapters, I was illustrating a very important tool/technique for handling the difficult subjects. The first one, the day that I left my Mother at the home in Colorado where she still resides, I was totally protected by the shock of my personal situation, post Hurricane Katrina. When Mom was angry and protested staying at the home I did not react at all. I sat with her, changed the subject, and told her I loved her. We talked about the pretty things in her room and waited until things were calm. I then attempted again to leave and finally I left as if we had not had the previous conversation and in her mind we had not—it is one of the few blessings of forgetfulness. We can only receive this blessing of forgetfulness, and it is more for them than for us, if we are willing to let anger and difficult periods pass and not try to justify/explain our actions and trying to get them to "bless us" with their approval. So often, we want to explain why they must do something that is not optional and is not their first choice, like staying in a 24-hour care center when that is the level of care they require. Then we want them not only to accept the decision they did not make but we want them to reassure us that they know we are making decisions in their best interest. While that is a wonderful idea, it is also irrational. What we need to strive toward is having good visits and departing on good terms which sometimes even means sneaking out when they are happily engaged with someone or something else.

It is so easy and so common, especially in the role of the primary caregiver—which I no longer held, to become very controlling, self-centered, guilt provoking and martyred! Please learn to watch your actions for such behavior; they will create untold problems with other family members and with the day center which is participating in your loved ones care. Most of all, it will create unnecessary concern and upheaval for the person with the disease. This was illustrated in a previous chapter when I grudgingly took my mother back to her home where she would have a proper dinner and go to bed early after an exhausting but pleasant day. She, as my mother, could sense I was upset and wanted to stay with me until I was comfortable. Consequently, she reached out for me and wanted to go with me, it was her responsibility. I, childishly, pulled her hands off of me, told her she couldn't go and hurried out the door; leaving her confused and defenseless and having erased the pleasantness of the entire day. This was clearly, all about me, not about her, which is why I was so upset. When I looked back and saw her forlornly waving I just wanted to dissolve into a little puddle!

It is so important to avoid these situations. The reason is about you as much as about them! I go back and forth repeatedly on this subject and it is often easier to use the child analogy. Would you take a 3 or a 5-year old out to dinner with a group of people at the end of a very busy and over-stimulating day? You know, if you do, the chances of anyone being able to enjoy the dinner will be slim. In addition, you are expecting the child to manage more than they are capable of managing. Now, there are parents who will subject their children to this situation; however, as they become more experienced they know better and plan better. It is the same situation with a person with dementia, they have limits on what they are able to do and enjoy and we have the responsibility to determine and set those limits. It is very difficult to stop including them in activities that they would have once enjoyed. However, they have a disease that has changed their capabilities. They need to have choices made in a way that manages that disease best.

I could have easily told my family that I wanted to stay and have dinner with Mom and I would meet with them afterward. However, that would likely have appeared as guilt provoking and martyrdom and it probably would have been that very thing. A more protective and mature choice would have been to take her home at a reasonable time and make sure she was comfortable. I could have spent time looking at all her pictures in her room, maybe even encouraged her to settle into her chair for a nap before dinner and then quietly slipped away. If she awoke, she would probably have thought she had a wonderful dream about being with her family—if she remembered the day at all. However, she would have had a pleasant evening with her friends and caregivers, without the trauma on either of our parts. In addition, I would have been able to have a nice dinner with the family and we would have enjoyed each other's company. It certainly would have prevented my panic every time I thought about our uncomfortable parting. Clearly, I had a choice but as caregivers we are so conditioned to self-blame that my experience is the perfect illustration of "what not to do" for this book.

Our story—from my perspective!

I can recount many stories in which I continued to want to be my mother's child; I wanted to be the one comforted, I wanted her gratitude for "all I was doing for her" and I wanted her blessing for all the choices that I needed to make. As a long distance caregiver I am very prone to thinking (fortunately I have enough experience to not act on this temporary insanity) what I would do if I were only with her. I am going to share my and Mom's experiences in this arena because I hope to illustrate the ludicrous thinking process we adopt as caregivers. We get so caught up in old roles and in the need for self justification we can make some very poor decisions and it creates a lot of unnecessary pain for everyone involved.

I tried for months to convince my Mom that she would be better off if she gave up her house and just lived with me. On occasion, she would even agree and then I would be furious when, "She acted as if we hadn't even had that conversation!" Did I simply forget that my mother was impaired or did I think she would selectively be able to put her disease 'on hold' to appease my emotional struggles?

Fortunately, in her Edith Bunker style of wisdom she finally got me to stop having those inane conversations when she asked why I did not use "my stuff" on her. When I replied that she was not demented, a fact I had obtusely chosen to deny, she brilliantly exclaimed, "You could be nice to me anyway."

I stressed myself to the max trying to "get home" earlier from work each day, as I was so concerned about her stress level when she would meet me at the door asking where I had been so long! I would justify, that I was earlier than I had told her and felt so unappreciated because I was "killing myself" to be her everything at all times—Why, did it take me so long to realize she wasn't capable of staying home alone!

When she finally, again in her sweet, simple and caring style, met me at the door as she and the dog, she had him on the leash, were headed out to see if I had been hurt, because she had heard an ambulance. Ambulances were something, you would hear hourly or more often, in the location we lived. At that point, I realized that something had to change—however, I assumed that her senior center hours of 9 A.M. to 3 P.M. would be adequate hours, regardless of the fact that she would then be home alone from 3 P.M. until I got home, until we could find a safer place to live, which took several months.

Then I determined that she had to go to the senior center, as she could not stay home alone all day. I should have introduced the new environment of the senior center for the day, as it really was, a way of life that was not optional. I went through some kind of a "half-baked" interview process and told Mom she would have a volunteer job. It took her no time at all to determine, she didn't want the job and she wasn't going. Why, when there was no option—did I treat it like there was? It is no wonder that she was so angry with me when I left her there. She loved that place, was always happy there, still often thinks that is where she is now as she talks about her job and the work she does almost daily. However, she fussed with me every day when we went there and told everyone for as long as she could that I "made her get a job and she didn't get paid!"

In our new home, which was a strain on the budget and not paid for by long-term care insurance, why did I think that she would be safe alone, again from 3:00 P.M. until I got home? Was it because she could not get out in the street and I had hidden the dog leash (which she always found)? I don't even want to tell you about the time she burnt up the dish in the microwave or the time she burned up the pan of hard boiled eggs she was cooking, in that new safe home. It was a miracle, for me that she stopped trying to cook after that; it certainly wasn't because I had her in the protected environment she required for her limitations.

In retrospect, I don't know why I didn't just have her stay at one of the homes where I worked after the senior center until time to go home. It would have been an easy, inexpensive solution and we would not have had to add the additional confusion of a move, they even delivered other people to those homes in the van, I wouldn't have had to pick her up and take her as I did when I took her home. Was it my fear of admitting that I couldn't do it all? In addition, I could have gone to Jazzercise at the end of the day, as I had prior to her moving in with me. She could have eaten at the home and I wouldn't have had to fix dinner every night. Even if I would have paid for that option, we could have used her long-term insurance to pay for it and it would have spared me additional expenses that I could ill afford and were obviously increasing my stress.

Last but certainly not least, when she became physically ill and the doctors felt it was unsafe for her to go to the senior center any longer—how could I possibly justify her staying at the house alone for three weeks until I moved her into one of the homes permanently. In her infinite wisdom, she pointed out to me, "I'm not alone because I have a perfectly good dog taking care of me!" How long would I have left her in a state of jeopardy?

Pain or Privilege?

As I have repeatedly pointed out in this book and in my presentations, we can't change history. However, we can learn from history so please learn from my history and do not make the same mistakes I made.

I made all the wrong decisions for all the right reasons and you too can fall into that caregiver trap! Understand this as a disease, so from your loved ones symptoms, seek a diagnosis and then develop a plan of care. It is your responsibility as the caregiver to follow that plan of care. Do it for the person with the disease, do not allow yourself to think that you are doing this to them or that they are "not ready" for a particular situation "yet".

There is pain and loss whenever there is illness. However, you do have a choice. You can accept the privilege of being the person who cares enough about the person who is ill, and selflessly outline and enact a plan to meet the needs of this regressive, degenerative illness. Alternatively, you can become obsessed with care giving and righteous indignation, deny the existence of the disease and severity, and place them in harms way. While the intent is noble the execution is flawed—please think and understand.

8

Never Falter
Always Persist

Never Falter: When they seem to have a good day or a lucid period, do not fall back into a state of denial and question if there has been a misdiagnosis. When the disease progresses, do not second guess what you have done to this point.

Always Persist: It is critical that you move forward, make the decisions that are in the best interest of your loved one and remember to take care of yourself. It is so easy to become emotional and irrational, but you must continue to move forward.

Now What Does That Mean?

It is best when symptoms appear to have an extensive evaluation and that should be the benchmark for at least an annual evaluation. The majority of the time, with this disease process, even the physicians are reluctant to provide the diagnosis. Denial is the overriding emotion on the part of everyone involved. It is astounding how consistently persons with a dementia diagnosis and the people who love them move backward and thus place the person who has the disease in harms way.

A good day in any disease process is a good day, nothing more nothing less. If one has cancer and they wake up feeling great, does it mean they don't have cancer? If a diabetic eats a piece of pie and has no reaction, does it mean they do not have diabetes? Learn to use the same rationale with a Dementia, regardless if it is caused from Alzheimers', Vascular, or some other disease process, appreciate and enjoy good days; do not deviate from the plan of care.

When things do not work out as planned, accept that it was a bad day, do not scrap the plan or accept the fact that "they refused" the new plan. If they complain, every day, as my mother did about going to the senior center, agree, do not explain, do not argue, just move forward and complete the plan. Stay out of the mix as much as possible. If you cannot handle moving forward then your responsibility will require having them picked up and delivered each day. You will be amazed at how many people will volunteer to provide that service, although you need to be willing to ask. Even if a friend cannot provide the service they often know someone who will be willing.

The idea that your loved one "is not ready for that yet" is very common and it is usually steeped in your inability to face their limitations. From the time of diagnosis it is critically important, for the person with the diagnosis, to develop a new daily routine that includes interaction with peers and provides an environment where they will feel useful and have a purpose in their life. So often, caregivers, take on the 24-hour care and somehow feel if people are clean, fed, clothed and in the company of their caregiver and "at home" their needs are met. Those needs are basic but the need for peers and a reason to be alive is critical to them for sustaining quality of life. If you find a situation (senior center, day care) depressing then find a situation that is better in your eyes. However, remember they have different capabilities than you have and certainly different than they once had. I know so many people who derived great pleasure by assisting persons who are more impaired than they were. Their families were worried that they would find the situation depressing but the opposite was usually the case. Do not expect the person with dementia to go ahead and look at a place and then say, "I would love to go there everyday or I would love to move there." That is not going to happen, even if it is true. Determine what is available, what you can afford (there are often resources, do not be reluctant to investigate), what is needed and then get started.

The worst possible situation is for a person with dementia is to stay at home, with no peers, no responsibility, no perceived need, just waiting to die—they will have a long, lonely and miserable wait.

I've used it before and I will use it again, don't forget the child analogy. Would you allow a kindergarten child to stay home because they don't like the school or simply because they don't want to go? I have seen mothers who try to plead and cajole and even threaten, to no avail; the situation just seems to get worse. If the mother isn't able to just move forward and leave them at the door, then the dad or a friend needs to take them to school and drop them off. Not attending school is rarely an option.

When you are the long distance caregiver, do not try to analyze, criticize or circumvent the process of arranging for the person with dementia to have a new daily routine in a protected and stimulating, for them, environment. It is very easy to give advice, so if you do not understand what is being done, be willing to spend money to have the situation professionally evaluated. There are professionals in every state called Geriatric Care Managers and they will, for a fee, do a professional evaluation of a situation and make recommendations for what is available in the community. Even if you are dealing with an "early onset" individual who would not be considered geriatric, Geriatric Care Managers are well trained to do this evaluation. If you truly disagree with what is being done be willing to follow the old adage, "Complaining makes one a volunteer". Ask what you can do to assist and then respond with the requested assistance not an unsolicited opinion.

Our story—from my perspective!

I have already shared, in previous chapters, our stories in respect to our daily routine as the primary caregiver. Even with twenty years experience and knowledge I obviously made some serious errors in judgment in respect to my Mother's care! I have had to learn to be the long distance caregiver and for the most part, I am able to manage this duty better. However, we probably should have a chapter inserted from my Sister and Brother who are now the "in State" caregivers. I am surmising that I do better because I now have the time to reevaluate all my "half-baked" ideas before attempting to implement them.

As the long distance caregiver I have two options for interacting with my Mom, the telephone and the visits.

We had one of those depressing phone calls. I called my Mom and she knew my voice before I could even say who I was. But it was downhill from there. She told me that someone had asked about her today and the old white haired woman said, "Oh, she doesn't know anything." Mom, understood and was humiliated but was stating that she could not do anything but just take it; she doesn't have anywhere else to go. I changed the subject and we talked about other things, she had gotten Christmas cards but she did not know who sent them, so I provided names to make conversation. I talked about what we had for dinner and the weather but she wanted me to come today so I could see her cards and take her with me! Then, suddenly she needed to go to the bathroom and she was concerned about the phone, and she said, "Who do I give this phone to? Well, I have to go now!" I knew intellectually that she was okay; she often remembered things people said about her and she could be very sensitive and sometimes thought people did not like her. Nothing has changed but I just felt so far away and I felt like I had abandoned her and she seemed so lost without me! I really understood why people stop calling their loved ones with dementia, but not calling truly made me feel worse. I am just so far away now and I still need and want those daily hugs. This just hurts, it makes my neck so tight, and I just miss her so much. This is just one of those many things in life through which one has to work. I want a fast forward button for our lives but then I know it has to get worse before it can get better and that is truly the worst thought!

You probably noticed that I have frequently vacillated from stating that I called every day, to thinking I can't ever call again, to calling every other day and to calling frequently. Initially, my calls really seemed to upset Mom and I did stop calling for a brief period of time especially when the phone just seemed to be confusing. I also realized that she couldn't talk on the phone when there were other people present. Initially, when I decided to stop calling Mom I told my sister. She was concerned about that decision so she would call me when she was visiting and could help Mom with the phone and that worked quite well. However, my sister's husband became ill and she was no longer able to visit often. Then I asked the staff about her schedule and now I call when she is in her room and not distracted by what is going on in the main room where they usually congregate.

In addition, I had to learn not to react to the conversation. For me, this was easy as it is something that I had trained people to do for years. Currently, I feel blessed with the phone conversations and I want to hang onto them forever. I probably average talking with Mom about five times a week, the calls last from 2-10 minutes. On occasion she truly seems to know who I am. Often, she is just her pleasant happy self and chats about many things. I just love the fact that I can hear her voice and tell her I love her, as I know I won't have that opportunity forever.

Pain or Privilege?

It is so easy to dwell on what might have been or how terribly unfair it can be when disease strikes. However, it is equally as easy to be grateful that your loved one with dementia is able to function without excruciating pain, is capable of conversing, and is still around for you to appreciate and hug. Disease does not 'play favorites'. Disease can happen to anyone and we can respond positively or negatively—the choice is ours.

For me, having Mom in the early years was my privilege. I sometimes made a mess of things; however, we truly enjoyed the majority of our time together and I have wonderful memories of those times. If I had it to do over again I would do things differently and ultimately would have not gotten as burned-out. For me, hindsight is 20-20 vision and for you perhaps my experience will provide you with that hindsight.

9

Never Quit
Always Expand

Never Quit: Often Alzheimer's is referred to as 'The Journey' because it is a process and it often lasts a long time. Regardless of the current situation, it is critical that you move forward with your own life and with theirs. Do not quit, continue to move forward.

Always Expand: Difficult times produce growth and learning, "It builds character." Like many things in life, "looking back, is much easier than living through it." Honestly, the only choice you have is how to "view" the journey. The "journey" is not optional.

Now What Does That Mean?

It takes all kinds of people to make up this world and thus it will take all kinds of people to be friends with a person with Alzheimer's disease or a related dementia. Consequently, there will be many ways of addressing the disease process. Some people just determine that they cannot handle it and bow out or essentially disappear. Others give it their entire life and thus disappear from an active life, away from the impaired loved one. Everyone tends to go from one side of the spectrum to the other as is common with all challenges. However, given some time and hopefully some education/information there is a way to find a 'happy medium' that is sustainable over whatever 'period of time' is required. This is one disease process that usually gives the caregiver enough time to eventually figure out the best way to manage it for his or her personality, for both the caregiver's and for the person for whom they are providing care. What it does not do is fix broken relationships. So often people say, "You would think now that we are dealing with this illness we could get along." Dealing with illness puts added stress on relationships; therefore, it is not logical to think it could fix broken relationships. It is much more likely to overstress the strong relationships, break the fragile ones, and create the opportunity to obliterate broken relationships. However, with some education and assistance from a support group, relationships can be forged, strengthened and rebuilt—as always, the choice is yours!

Our story—from my perspective!

I just believed that if we just did not change our life patterns then the disease would "not get worse". I also believed that regardless of the disease, my Mom was capable of doing the things we had always done, "because she enjoyed them." Now, intellectually, I knew that even if it is something as simple as the "common cold", when someone does not feel well he or she automatically reduce his or her activity. However, even as the 'dementia expert' who constantly advised that "structure" was important, I continued to throw my Mom into stressful change situations. My reasons were sound; I truly did not want her to miss anything. My logic was flawed as I did not look at it from her perspective. No, I looked at it from her "before disease" perspective, but that was no longer reality.

The last trip we took, prior to the Hurricane Katrina evacuation was truly a nightmare. I had always prided myself on spending each of my grandsons birthday's with them. Mom loved birthday celebrations and children, so naturally I thought that she would enjoy those trips. My oldest grandson's birthday is July 5 and in 2005, as usual, I planned our trip to Chicago for his birthday. Funds were increasingly tight with all the changes that I had made for Mom to live with me. Consequently, I found this inexpensive flight from New Orleans to Chicago that made it more affordable. However, it was not a non-stop flight, which would be more difficult for Mom. I comforted myself with the idea that we would have airport assisted service and she would be in a wheelchair so it would not matter. I want to digress here to tell you how previously the wheelchair assistance had been going. Because of Mom's heart condition the doctors had said she should not walk long distances as she became too winded and could go into cardiac arrest. I had been requesting wheel chair assistance so we could travel without putting her at risk. She has always looked very young for her age and she looked healthy as well. We would get to the airport and when they would come with the wheel chair she would tell them that she did not need the chair. I would tell them that she did and she would continue to tell them and anyone else who would listen, like the TSA people in the security line and other people in line, that she did not need the wheelchair. She would say,

"I do not need this chair give it to someone else," and would then look at me and say why don't you ride in this chair. She truly didn't look like she needed the chair but I was just able to "live with it" and knew better than to try to correct her! Now, back to the trip, it was July and we encountered some extremely bad weather so we couldn't land at the destination airport. In fact, we had to go around it and we got into such extreme turbulence that the plane actually dropped. I've traveled a lot, for years, and it was without a doubt the roughest ride I've ever had. We then had to stop at another airport on the UPS runway to refuel and wait until the skies cleared as our destination airport had been temporarily closed. Thus, several hours later we arrived at the airport and had to wait in long lines. Instead of getting to Chicago at 8:00 P.M. we were in line in North Carolina at 9:00 P.M. and on our way to a hotel to spend the night at 10:30 P.M. We did not have clothing, no medication for Mom, and we hadn't eaten since lunch. I was pushing her in the airport wheel chair as the attendants were all busy. We got to the hotel but their kitchen was closed and they let us borrow an old wheelchair (with the rubber missing from one wheel) to go to the nearest restaurant several parking lots away. I was trying to push Mom in this broken wheelchair and get her over curbs and she was tired and just wanted to walk. In retrospect, it seems somewhat humorous but at the time it wasn't. We finally got to the restaurant, ate, and got back to our room to sleep. We had to sleep in our clothing and then get up quite early to catch the shuttle to get back to the airport. Mom was less than pleased with the entire mess and she just kept asking me, "Where we were going and why couldn't we just go home?" We finally got to Chicago about noon the next day and Mom was confused and exhausted. We hadn't been at my son's house very long and I noticed my two little grandsons's sliding along the wall very quietly! I asked them what they were doing and they said "Shh! She will hear us!" I said, "Who will hear you?" They said, "Shh! Great Grandma Honey!" About that time Mom came around the corner and said, "There they are, catch them that big one and the little one are tearing up this hotel and we can't even afford to stay here!" Therefore, you see that was how much she was enjoying our trip and it probably is no surprise to you that the next week she was back in the hospital with heart problems again. I just wanted her to be a part of my life and the life she once enjoyed, however, that was no longer feasible or even safe.

Fortunately, I got the picture and intellectually understood. However, I did try to convince myself if we hadn't had bad weather she wouldn't have been so tired etc. It did make it somewhat easier to accept the fact that she probably wasn't going to be able to make the birthday trips again. Now, I still planned to take her home for Christmas!

Then life intervened. As I shared earlier, I had placed Mom in one of the homes that I had implemented in New Orleans. Then, with the approach of Hurricane Katrina, we evacuated those homes, Mom was with me and the other 25 residents and 12 staff from those homes. We were on the road and in strange places. Mom was less than happy with me. She kept asking me, "What have you done to get us kicked out of our home?" She just wanted to go back to her own little home that she liked so much and stop traveling around and she certainly wanted no part of sleeping on air mattresses on the floor. There was something worse than an air mattress, when we offered her a cot she was truly insulted. She was the same Mom who would never have complained about anything no matter what she had to encounter. With the disease process things had obviously changed, because of the "frontal lobe" impairment she was saying exactly what she was thinking. My mild mannered mother had lost some of her meekness and she was truly exasperated with the entire traveling situation.

Nearly a month later, after my responsibility for taking care of the other residents was complete, we arrived back at my son's in Chicago. He hadn't really noticed the progression of the disease process in July but now in late September especially after traveling for a month he clearly stated that the person with me was not the Grandma he knew. Here is a story, as told by my son about an incident that will last in his mind forever.

"Grandma just tried to kill me! I truly mean it." I told my Mom, Jo, that she and Grandma could come and live with me—in fact, I bribed my Mom so that they would come. They were Hurricane Katrina victims who had both lost their homes and I had a nice home in a Chicago suburb certainly out of the path of Hurricanes. They would be safe and Mom could expand her small business and I could help her with Grandma—but Mom left to run some errands and Grandma almost killed me. Well maybe I am exaggerating a little but she did nearly knock me off a ladder and I would have fallen 15 feet. Grandma was sleeping on the couch so Mom said she was going to run a few errands. It was my weekend without the boys and I was painting the entryway in my home. It required an extension ladder and I had it safely balanced against the top window. I was putting the blue masking tape around the window so it wouldn't get paint splatter. I will admit I had my IPOD on so I couldn't hear anything. All of a sudden the ladder started swinging—I am not exaggerating. I hung on for dear life and looked down and Grandma was shaking the ladder with both hands. I could tell she was shouting but I couldn't let go of the ladder with either hand as I was teetering on the brink of really falling as she was still shaking the ladder and I looked like a cartoon character. I grabbed the window frame and yelled "Grandma Stop." She looked stricken but let go of the ladder. I pulled my IPOD out of my ears as I scurried safely down the ladder. I was out of control and I yelled, "Grandma why were you trying to knock me off the ladder?" She said, "I told you not to paint that nice white paint blue, it is ugly". Now I truly had to laugh because my Grandma would never say anything bad about anything so I told her that it wasn't paint it was tape and I would take it off after I painted." Grandma always loved to paint so I told her all about the paint I was putting on the wall and showed her the color and she seemed totally content and happy. I even got her a cup of coffee and got her all settled. She always used to just sit and smile, she was just the best Grandma in the world it was always "all about us". I foolishly got right back on the ladder because time is so precious to me and I had so much to do. Of course put my IPOD back in my ears and I just got to the top, when Grandma was swinging that ladder again. However, this time when I yelled, she just shook the ladder harder—it looked like she was going to succeed in knocking me off! I held on to the wall and tried to pretend I was on a carnival ride but Grandma was determined to get me off that ladder! I kept yelling "Grandma! Stop!" but that just made her more determined. Thankfully, my Mom walked in, went over to Grandma, and led her away. I shakily got down and asked Mom why Grandma was trying to kill me and Grandma answered, "That man is ruining our woodwork, you need to fire him, and he won't stop when I tell him to!" It was not funny, though Mom and Grandma laughed and laughed. I told Grandma that I was not painting the woodwork, I was protecting it and she just told Mom that she needed to fire me! Somehow, I had gone from her darling grandson, who could do no wrong, to an incompetent painter whom she wanted fired and Grandma would never have fired anyone—especially if he or she were incompetent. I was going to have to rescind my offer for them to live with us; I could not have Grandma living with us if she was going to try to kill me! I told Mom I would pay $500 on the spot if there were a way I could understand what was going on with Grandma and how to manage her effectively. Grandma had a 5-minute attention span and she did not believe a thing I told her—this was not my Grandma and we could not live this way.

Pain or Privilege?

Pain, well the pain was really present for both my children and my grandchildren. What seemed like my choice at the time, was to choose between my mother, my children and my grandchildren. It was, finally, obvious that Mom was no longer able to travel and she was not enjoying the trips anyway. In addition, the children didn't understand her and she didn't even recognize them. Now if they came to visit, when she was not taxed by fatigue and change, she would enjoy them and they could retain good memories of her. In my children's living environment it was to difficult for both my Mom and the children. I realized this in July but I truly thought I had until Christmas to make plans for the management of this situation.

Then our lives changed forever. It was almost as if I had forgotten that Mom was absolutely thriving in her 24-hour care home. I went back to thinking that she could just fit into our environment so I could take care of her. I have to be grateful to Mom for making it very clear that my son's lifestyle and his home were just not a place where my Mom would be comfortable. In addition, my family felt it best that she be back in her own community where friends and relatives could visit. Fortunately, for me, the decision was taken out of my hands. I was in no position to make a decision at that time of upheaval in my life and quite frankly I would not have made an appropriate decision anyway. As I have suggested from the beginning of this book to the end, my zeal to take care of my mother, somehow prevented me from making rational decisions that were in her best interest.

It has truly been my privilege to have the opportunity to spend so much quality time with my Mom in my lifetime. I know few people who have had the amount of time, as adults, with a parent. I am so richly blessed that she has been such a joy and of course it is very difficult to let go of that time and attention. It has been particularly difficult as I have also experienced so much loss at this stage of my life. Ultimately, I will be able to focus on the wonderful privilege of the time with my Mother and hopefully forget the pain.

10

Never Despair
Always Enjoy

Never Despair: I am not trying to minimize the devastation of this disease process. However, I am trying to point out some ways to avoid the absolute despair it can cause.

Always Enjoy: There are so many things that are truly enjoyable about a person for whom you care. Rarely, are those things remembered in terms of the stimulating conversations. Usually, they are about the times you have shared and the ability to enjoy what time we have left together.

Now What Does That Mean?

This is one of those things in life that seems contradictory. I have always found such things easier to understand if you can think of them as 'full circle' instead of opposite ends of a continuum. The entire theme of this book, I am saying, "It isn't about you," and then I am saying, "It is about you." When it comes to making decisions in your loved one's best interest it has to be about them not about you. When it comes to taking care of yourself it is about you. However, taking care of yourself does not include postponing your life and dedicating your life to their care. The result of that level of dedication is high stress that promotes self-neglect, ultimate illness and perhaps even death.

Now, in this chapter, I am saying don't be devastated instead enjoy the person. Now how can you possibly enjoy a person who for all real purposes, certainly in the roles you have shared in life, no longer exists? If you can learn to enjoy this precious person, just as they are; you will always be grateful. If you just cannot enjoy being with them, then perhaps it just was not meant to be.

Our story—from my perspective!

Mom and I are having wonderful conversations these days! I truly wonder what the staff, where she lives, thinks of the conversations as they often hear them from Mom's side. I am so grateful for all my years of training because I really know how to have these conversations and I am able to do it! Now, it isn't always easy and some days I feel elated after I talk to her and other days I feel very sad. However, I have had both wonderful and horrible visits with my Mom so now whatever happens seems almost normal.

In some conversations I feel certain she doesn't have any idea who I am but she is very cheerful. Other days I know she knows exactly who I am because she asks about my ex-husband (of 30 years) by name and wants to know if he is there or still mad at me! Other days she is in a wonderful world. She tells me all the things she has done and she clearly is sharing the story of the day in her life, which must be her favorite time of her life. She has her four little children and she is helping Dad on the farm. Apparently, she acts out those days using dolls and stuffed animals for the children. Some days she is busy at her job and she has worked all day and it is at a Church or a School, which makes me smile and feel forgiven. You see, the senior center where I took her everyday for several years was in a church and she always called it school. She has never worked in a Church or a School so, for me, I feel certain she is in that center and she is happy. Then there are those very rare days when she is very lucid. The other day she even told me that, when no one is looking she sometimes plays with her stuffed animals and pretends they are we kids when we were little.

I have counseled people over the years about not expecting too much, but to focus on the importance of enjoying the time together. I have a dear friend whose Mom for a number of years was in one of the homes I ran. In the early days, he picked her up every Sunday morning, took her to Mass, and took her to his house to spend the day. They had difficult times, on occasion, but as a whole the days were great and he really enjoyed her and their time together. He was able to enjoy her wherever she was in her disease process and she did have some very difficult days.

Eventually, she developed very serious heart problems (almost exactly the same as the heart problems my mother has) and she just could not tolerate going to church. So he would take her to his house. Eventually, that became too difficult and he asked me what he should do. I said, "Just visit her at the house and don't try to take her out anymore." That was really difficult for him as he wanted to spend the time together, he wanted her to be around his children (though they had stopped enjoying those days) and he didn't want to feel like he was abandoning her. He really loved his Mom so he started coming to spend part of every Sunday at the house. He would cook for everyone and his outing for his Mom was to take her for a ride around the block in the wheel chair. She enjoyed those visits and so did he. In addition, he developed an even greater appreciation for how truly incredible was our staff.

His Mom just beamed when he walked in the door and she would introduce him as her son long after she was able to articulate anything else accurately. He carried this process of enjoying her to the last days of her life. When we were certain that she was in her last hours he would go to work, go to dinner and do homework with his daughter and then come and spend the night with his Mom. He would sit beside her bed, hold her hand and tell her how wonderful she was and always had been to him. She rarely responded those 5 or 6 days but he was there and he was faithful to her. I don't know that I have ever seen anything more beautiful or touching in my life. I sat with them for an hour or so the evening she died. He finally told me to leave and go take care of my own Momma who was eating dinner with the other people in the home. The staff called shortly after I left to say she had passed. I, of course, left Momma Home with the Dog and went back to provide comfort. However, it wasn't necessary because he had provided his own comfort by enjoying her even to her last breath. He still calls me every Mother's Day to thank me for providing a way for him to take care of his Momma—what an honor for me!

Now let me share the story of another man and the visit he had with his Mom. However, there is another scenario, which I will describe, with just a few changes that show the potential for the same visit to be good rather than devastating. The visits are the same visit the difference is Despair or Enjoy:

Scenario 1—the real visit—despair!

I am Tom and this was a Christmas visit that was just awful, it hurt more than you can ever imagine anything could hurt! Mom did not even look like herself, she looked slightly disheveled and what was wrong with her eye, it was almost bloody looking and her face did not use to sag like that, did it, her lipstick was all crooked and she looked like a clown? I had no idea what to say when she looked at me and asked if I had seen Tom. I am Tom but no amount of repetition of that fact even stopped her repeated question "Have you seen my son, Tom?" She always loved presents and it felt a little better for a moment as she gleefully tore into her present. Then she held the new pajamas to her face and said "What a nice kitten." I just had to get out of there! I had planned to spend several hours but now after 10 minutes into the visit, I just had to go! That wasn't my Mom and no one should have to live that way! I left just wanting to cry. I had driven for several hours to see her and just could not stay and visit. I do not even think I hugged her and I really do not know if I can go back! What on earth is the disease that destroys the person like this, wouldn't it be better for everyone if she were in heaven with dad? Now I have said it out loud, it seems that the only way this can get better if for it to get worse, much worse, how can I possibly actually wish she were gone. There ought to be a way to manage this that is better for her and yes for me too!

Scenario 2—How it could be—enjoy!

What if you could have the Christmas visit you had always envisioned? To see the recognition in her eyes and you came up to her and hugged her—she hugged you so tight and said "I knew it was you when you came in". She looked so cute in her Christmas outfit, she didn't look nearly as bad as I had anticipated, the blood in her eye was almost gone and her attempts at being all fancy was so cute—almost like she was playing dress-up, her lipstick was crooked but she had clearly done it herself . She grabbed at the present and tore it open, again just like a child, she loved the softness so much she held it comfortingly to her face and petted it like a kitten. She had always loved cats so much so I knew she liked it because she compared it to an all time love. She seemed so content and happy and she couldn't sit still for a minute, she kept getting up, going away, and then coming back. I asked her where she was going and she said, "I have a job, I am checking on things, I can't just sit here and do nothing like some people!" Normally, Mom would never have said anything feisty, she was queen of, "if you don't have anything nice to say, don't say anything at all". I sort of like her spunk and she truly believes that she is needed here, she even has a job. That is so much better than sitting in a chair all droopy and forlorn or even worse sleepy and drooling! It is so wonderful not to envision her, sitting in a chair in her only half of the room! She just owns this whole place and even runs it and it seems perfectly o.k. with the people who run the place, too. I had so much to do today and it was just great that I could visit for a short time and then leave. I told her I had to go and of course the moment I dreaded came she asked to go with me! I got a sad look on my face and she started getting sad too as I hugged her—she might not act like a Mom but boy she can still read my body language. Then one of those angels who helps to take care of her came up and said, "Aren't you going to come and help us with lunch?" She changed posture in a second, let go of me, headed off happily being useful and needed and I was forgotten—or as we used to say "thrown under the bus!" There are some real advantages to her not being oriented to time, though she probably didn't know my name or even that I was her son—she knew that I was there to visit her. She is very content with her life, she loved seeing me but I know that as often as I see her it is enough because she has a life—did not she say it herself, " she can't just sit around like some people".

Pain or Privilege?

I've shared earlier in this book that there were times when I just couldn't even call my Mom because the calls were so distressing. However, my son, the same one who believes that Mom tried to "kill him" asked me why I was distressed after the calls. He said, "It sounds to me like Grandma is very happy, just be happy with her." Now, that should have been obvious, especially to me the "expert" but it wasn't until I heard it out loud. So, I am writing it "out loud" for you to see and hear in case it isn't obvious to you

What I am also telling you is that you can and should visit, but it only has to be as often as you need to justify to yourself so that you will not feel guilty. The entire Pain and Pleasure scenario that I have depicted is illustrated in this chapter. You have a choice about how you react to this and how you view it, in your mind. It is the proverbial, "Cup half empty, cup half full," the cup is the same it is how each individual perceives the cup that is open to interpretation.

In my years of experience I have felt the most sympathy for the spouses and children who just could not bring themselves to call or visit. They don't get the distinct advantage of working through the grief and loss. Unfortunately, when the person is gone they tend to live with a lot of regret. They say, "It is a blessing," but they do not seem to have the peace that the person who has been able to enjoy their loved one through the disease process to the end.

Whatever you choose, whether you go "kicking and screaming and pushing yourself every inch of the way", or embrace the illness and choose to "look at it in an entirely different light and enjoy what is left," or "just don't go and try not to think about them too often." The choice is yours to make and ultimately that choice will be the one that you have to live with for the rest of your life. However, please remember your loved one loves you and they do not want you to be miserable. Regardless of how you choose to manage the disease process of your loved one, please, "take it easy on yourself", be good to yourself." This entire process will always be one of the most difficult processes of your entire life! There is no other statement that I have seen to be consistently true in my twenty plus years experience in this field.

Conclusion

Choice is a wonderful thing unless it feels as if you have no choice! Caregiver's of persons with Alzheimer's disease or a related dementia often feel that they have no choice. When it comes to the disease, that feeling is accurate. However, when it comes to how one can manage quality of life, for both the caregiver and the one afflicted with the disease, there are a lot of choices. In fact, the choice is yours; you can proceed with pain or with pleasure.

I hope that sharing my mother and my stories has provided you a basis for inserting your own stories. You can experience the triumphs and frustrations, the good times and the bad times. You can see the opportunity for practicing new skills and using new tools. Ultimately, you can choose to perceive things differently and make choices that are truly in the best interest of the one for whom you care. It is "all about you" in the perspective that your ultimate responsibility is that you must take care of yourself so you will remain in good health and available to "look out for them" even if someone else provides the physical care. However, it is "not about you" when it comes to decisions, as the decisions need to be for them and what serves them best, continually taking their disease and it is limitations into account.

Quality of life is difficult to measure. However, when it comes to a person with Dementia, (regardless of what is causing that brain degeneration) measure quality of life by what your loved one sees as worth and purpose in their daily life. It may seem boring and repetitive to us but for them it is their quality of lifeline! It is never too early to enroll them in a day center. Initially, they can go as a volunteer and segue into a participant role as time passes. Do not expect to get permission, approval or a thank you for the changes you orchestrate into their lives. Move forward to address their need for self-worth and purpose regardless of what they might be "insisting upon" or "refusing" to do. This is information that applies only to someone who truly has a dementia diagnosis. Obtaining that diagnosis is also critical and requires a complete neurological work-up not just an opinion.

Resources, both physical and financial, are very difficult for the majority of persons to access and to accept. However, it just requires tenacity on the part of the caregiver to find these services. Do not ever assume that you can do this alone, get in a support group and listen to what others in that group are telling you. Do not assume that you can or even should be the only one who cares for your loved one or you will indeed "put them and yourself, in harms way." Start with Associations and Foundations, at the very least access the Alzheimer's Association and/or Alzheimer's Foundation, AARP, and the Area Agency on Aging. If you do not have internet access, then check the yellow pages, go to the Library and ask for assistance. Do not take 'no' for an answer; if you cannot find answers, call back the next day and talk to a different person. Often, volunteers answer the phones and some days you will get more information than on other days. Many communities have Senior Resource Guides and they are an excellent tool to use when making calls. If someone does not have a particular service available, ask if he or she knows of someone who might be of assistance. Take notes and keep calling.

Last, but certainly not least. Do not get so busy providing care that you forget why and for whom you care. Early on in this disease process, the person with Dementia will lose some level of communication and ultimately even the role you have played in their life, you won't necessarily be their daughter/son or husband/wife. However, they will recognize that you belong to them; they know they love you and they will respond to smiles, hugs, touch and basic kindness to the very end. Learn to "let go" of the role they provided to the community and even in your life. Work on appreciating them for the living, breathing human being they are today and appreciate the fact that you can hear their voice, see their smile and touch their hand. Ultimately, what is important in life is life itself and when you can hang onto that fact, the journey will become much easier and even more rewarding.

Thank you for sharing this journey with me and with your loved one. It is my fondest hope that in some way this story will make your journey easier.

About the Author

Jo Huey has worked with persons with Alzheimer's disease since 1986. She has a Certificate in Gerontology from the University of Denver and a Master of Social Science from the University of Colorado. Jo, a Native of Colorado moved to New Orleans in 1997. She has two grown children, a daughter and a son, and three grandsons.

TEN ABSOLUTES
ABSOLUTELY NEVER!!!!!!!!

1. ARGUE	instead	AGREE
2. REASON	instead	DIVERT
3. SHAME	instead	DISTRACT
4. LECTURE	instead	REASSURE
5. SAY "REMEMBER"	instead	REMINISCE
6. SAY "I TOLD YOU"	instead	REPEAT/REGROUP
7. SAY "YOU CAN'T"	instead	DO WHAT THEYCAN
8. COMMAND/DEMAND	instead	ASK/MODEL
9. CONDESCEND	instead	ENCOURAGE/PRAISE
10. FORCE	instead	REINFORCE

ISBN 142512705-3

9 781425 127053

Edwards Brothers Malloy
Thorofare, NJ USA
July 17, 2015